Cast Iron Technology

Volume 1

Cast Iron Technology

Volume 1

Dr. S.N. Tiwari
B.Sc. (Met. Engg.), M.Sc. (Met. Engg.), Ph.D. (Met. Engg.)
Director, Moradabad Institute of Technology
Ex-Professor & Head, Department of Metallurgical Engineering, and Ex-Coordinator of Centre of Advanced Study in Metallurgy, Institute of Technology, Banaras Hindu University
Ex-Dean, Faculty of Engineering & Technology, Banaras Hindu University

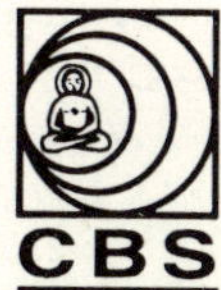

CBS PUBLISHERS & DISTRIBUTORS PVT. LTD.
New Delhi • Bangalore • Pune • Cochin • Chennai (India)

Soft Cover ISBN : 978-81-239-1489-3
Hard Cover ISBN : 978-81-239-1496-1

First Edition : 2007
Reprint : 2010

Published by Satish Kumar Jain and produced by V.K. Jain for
CBS Publishers & Distributors Pvt. Ltd.,
CBS Plaza, 4819/XI Prahlad Street, 24 Ansari Road, Daryaganj,
New Delhi - 110002, India. • Website: www.cbspd.com
e-mail: delhi@cbspd.com, cbspubs@vsnl.com, cbspubs@airtelmail.in
Ph.: 23289259, 23266861, 23266867 • Fax: 011-23243014

Branches:

- ***Bangalore:*** Seema House, 2975, 17th Cross, K.R. Road, Bansankari 2nd Stage, Bangalore - 560070 Ph.: 26771678/79 Fax: 080-26771680 • e-mail: bangalore@cbspd.com
- ***Pune:*** Shaan Brahmha Complex, 631/632, Basement, Appa Balwant Chowk, Budhwar Peth, Next to Ratan Talkies, Pune - 411002 Ph.: 020-24464057/58 • Fax: 020-24464059 e-mail: pune@cbspd.com
- ***Cochin:*** 36/14, Kalluvilakam, Lissie Hospital Road, Cochin - 682018, Kerala • e-mail: cochin@cbspd.com Ph.: 0484-4059061-65 • Fax: 0484-4059065
- ***Chennai:*** 20, West Park Road, Shenoy Nagar, Chennai - 600030 e-mail: chennai@cbspd.com Ph.: 044-26260666-26202620 Fax: 044-45530020

Printed at :
India Binding House, Noida (UP)

Dedicated to My Parents

Preface

Cast irons are the tonnage product of the foundry industry and represent more than 80% of the cast metals produced. Unfortunately, there is hardly any text book which deals with all aspects of such an important engineering hardware including production technology, metallurgy, properties and applications of all members of a large family of cast irons at one place. The information available in literature is scattered and sometimes confusing and presented in parts in several publications.

It is the endevour of this author to fill up this existing gap by providing sufficient information on all above aspects of cast irons at one place under the book heading of Cast Iron Technology based on a through survey of exiting published knowledge, data and information. The author had designed in past a comprehensire course on cast iron technology and has taught different aspects of this course at the undergraduate and postgraduate levels for the last four decades. He is therefore hopeful that such a textbook or reference material will be very useful to students and teachers of all the engineering institutions besides the actual plant operators and users of the iron castings.

This book is divided into two parts and consists of a total of fifteen chapters. The first part of the book consists of eight chapters dealing with introduction and classification of cast irons, their melting practice with particular reference to developments in cupola melting practice, metallurgy, production technology, characterization and applications of all important family members of cast irons including gray cast irons, white and maleable cast irons, spheroidal graphite cast irons, vermicular (compacted) graphite cast irons and high-duty cast irons. It also provides the relevant references of all above chapters as a last section of this part of the book.

The second part of this book deals with the science of production and characterization of special (high-alloy) cast irons, selection of cast irons for different engineering applications, defects of iron castings and their remedies, welding of cast irons, inspection and testing as well as design of iron castings and finally, the Indian practice of cast iron technology. At the end, it will also include both the subject and the author indices besides the relevant references of the different chapters.

This book has been also written with a view to encourage advanced research in the areas of cast iron technology by providing the latest available in literature.

Any suggestions by the readers meant to improve the contents of this book shall be most welcome and greatly appreciated by the author.

June 2006 **S. N. Tiwari**

VARANASI

Acknowledgements

At the outset, I would like to thank the All India Council of Technical Education, New Delhi for providing me the financial assistance in the form of Emeritus Fellowship and the contigency grant to enable me to prepare the required manuscript of this book. It is my duty to express my most sincere thanks and gratitude to all the authors/editors/publishers of the books/monographs/ research papers etc. contained in the "List of References" as well as cited along with the figures whose figures/photomicrographs have been reproduced and whose work has been frequently consulted and quoted in the compilation of the Part I and II of the present book.

I am also thankful to many of my colleagues and friends, particularly Professor S.N. Upadhyay, the Director of the Institute of Technology, B.H.U. and Professor R.C. Gupta, the Head of Department of Metallurgical Engineering, I.T., B.H.U. for encouraging me in this endevour and providing the library and other departmental facilities and Dr. P. Sriram, my classmate and presently the Joint Managing Director of Rapsree Engineering Industries Ltd., Bangalore and Shri D.P. Upadhyaya, a very close friend of mine and Ex-Chief Metallurgist, Hindustan Mortors, Hoogly for their guidance and moral support. I am also thankful to one of my students, Shri Upendra Kumar for helping me in preparing and compilation of the diagrams and photomicrographs as a part of this book. My thanks are also due to Shri Vidya Shankar Singh for his patient and careful computer typing of the manuscript of this book.

S.N. Tiwari

BRIEF CONTENTS OF CAST IRON TECHNOLOGY
VOL-I

VOL-II

Contents

Cast Irons—Concepts, Terminology and Classification

1.1 INTRODUCTION

Cast irons are among the most popular and common engineering materials characterized with a wide range of mechanical properties of strength, hardness and ductility, machinability, wear, abrasive and corrosion resistance as well as very good foundry properties. They are the tonnage product of the foundry industry. It is said that out of 5 tons of castings produced, every 3 tons are that of cast irons. Cast irons also represent the largest tonnage of ferrous castings produced in the world. The reason for their popularity are that they are the cheapest ferrous alloys that can be easily melted and cast and it is possible to achieve diverse combinations of properties, extremely hard and brittle at one hand and soft, ductile and machinable at the other.

Cast irons represent a family of materials and not just one material which vary widely in their properties. Metallurgically, they are primarily alloys of iron, carbon and silicon which also contain significant amounts of manganese, phosphorus and sulfur and occasionally, other alloying elements like Ni, Cr, Mo and V

1.2 TERMINOLOGY AND DEFINITIONS

The term CAST IRON refers to a wide range of iron-carbon-silicon alloys containing upto 4% carbon and upto about 3.5% silicon in combination with varying percentages of manganese, sulfur and phosphorus as impurities. They are ordinarily, not usefully ductile as cast. In terms of iron-carbon phase diagram, cast irons are alloys of iron and carbon containing amounts of carbon in excess of the amount which can be retained in solid solution in austenite i.e.

irons containing more than 2 percent of carbon. Cast irons differ from steels in that they may contain free carbon (graphite) whereas steels do not. Further, steels can be obtained in both the forged and cast conditions whereas, most cast irons are available in cast conditions only.

The following are some six basic components of the family of cast irons.

1.2.1 Gray Cast Irons

They are the irons having a chemical composition such that after freezing a part or whole of its carbon occurs in the cast structure as free or graphitic carbon in the "flake form". On fracture such cast irons always present a gray sooty surface (the presence of the free carbon darkens the fracture) and therefore, known as gray irons. Such irons are highly brittle but have the lowest casting temperature, the least shrinkage and the best castability of all ferrous metals. The flakes of graphite are found to be distributed through out the matrix of the cast structure which may be ferrite, ferrite plus pearlite or pearlite depending upon the composition and the cooling rate prevailing during freezing. Fig. 1.1 shows typically the cast structure of such irons.

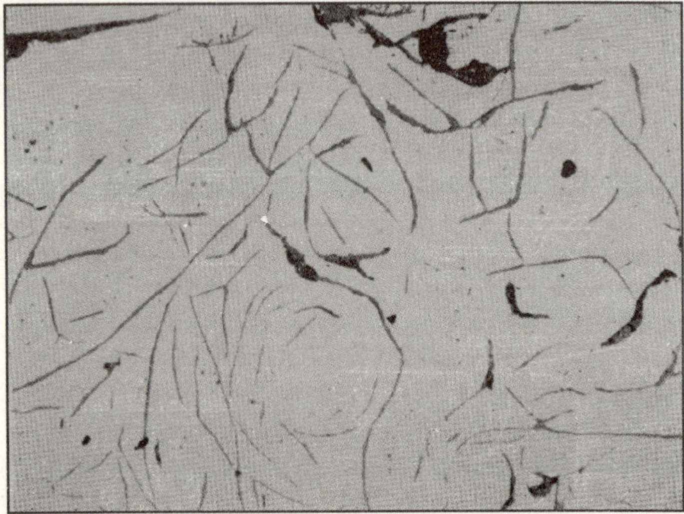

Fig. 1.1: Gray cast iron showing coarse graphite flakes in matrix of ferrite, X150. (From *Applied Science in the Casting of Metals* (ed. K. Strauss), Pergamon Press, Oxford, 1970, p. 187)

1.2.2 White Cast Irons

They are the irons having a chemical composition such that after freezing all of its carbon is found to be present in chemically combined form as cementite (Iron carbide, Fe_3C). Such irons are very hard and unmachinable and on fracture, present a white crystalline surface and therefore, known as white irons. They are characterized with very high abrasive resistance. The cast structure of such irons shows presence of massive cementite in the matrix of pearlite and is virtually free from any graphitic carbon as shown in Fig. 1.2.

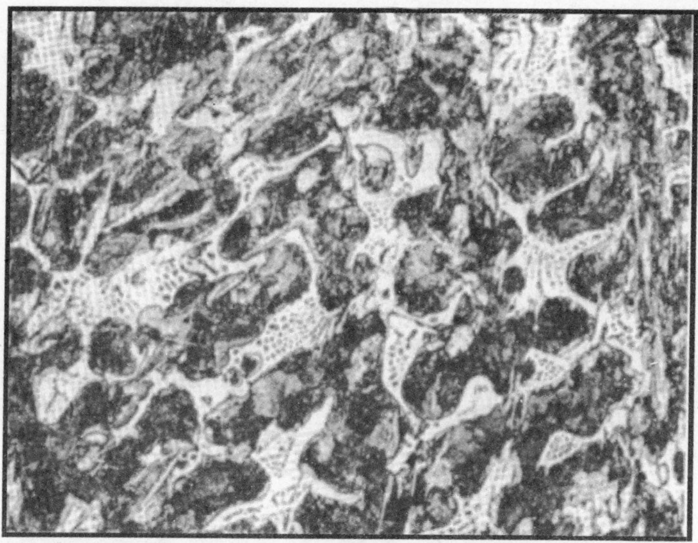

Fig. 1.2: White cast iron showing massive cementites in matrix of pearlite, X150 (Courtesy of Portcullis Press, Redhill).

Chilled Cast Irons: They are the irons of such composition which would normally freeze as gray cast irons but they are caused to freeze as white cast irons in some locations subjected to rapid cooling i.e. chilling during freezing. Such irons have high surface wear and abrasion resistance. The fractured surfaces of chilled cast irons show areas of white iron where freezing was fast and other areas of gray iron where the cooling rate was normal or slow.

1.2.3 Mottled Irons

They are the cast irons of the border line composition between the gray and white cast irons and freeze partly as a white cast iron and partly as gray cast irons under prevailing cooling conditions. Figure 1.3 shows a typical structure of such irons.

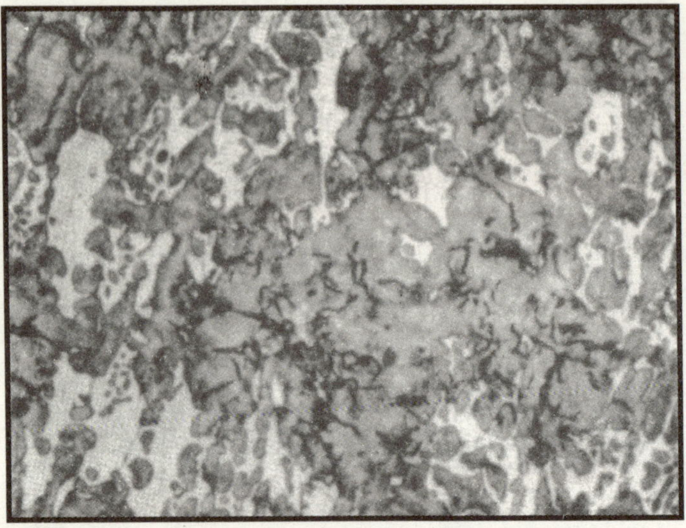

Fig. 1.3: Mottled iron showing both graphite and cementite in matrix of pearlite, X100 (Reprinted with permission of ASM International).

1.2.4 Malleable Irons

They are the cast irons of white iron compositions but characterized with good ductility or malleability produced by heat treating their castings of suitable chemical compositions. A part or whole of the carbon of such irons occurs in the free state as nodular-shaped aggregates of graphite. Such forms of compact graphite is also known as temper carbon which has the shape of rosette or nodule. Figure 1.4 shows a typical structure of such malleable irons.

1.2.5 Nodular or Spheroidal Graphite (S.G.) Irons

These are the specially prepared irons treated in the molten condition with a small percentage of magnesium, cerium or other agent which causes a large proportion of their carbon to occur as spheroids of graphite rather than flakes in the cast structure. Such irons are characterized with good ductility combined with high

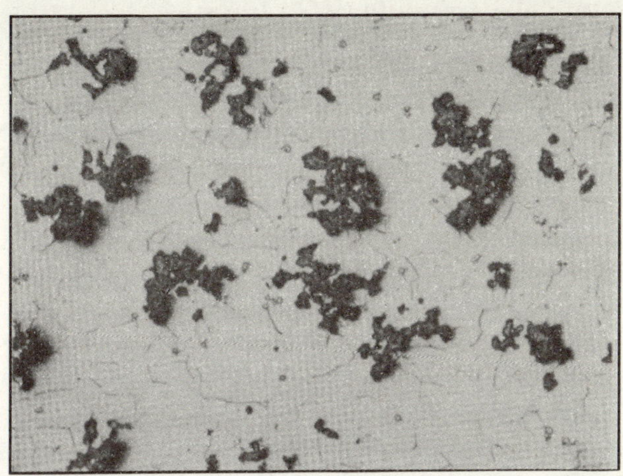

Fig. 1.4: Malleable iron showing graphite aggregates in matrix of ferrite, X150 (Courtesy of Portcullis Press, Redhill).

strength and therefore, such irons are also called as DUCTILE IRONS. On fracture, such irons present a bright steely surface. The globular shaped graphite is found to be distributed in a matrix of ferrite, ferrite plus pearlite or pearlite in the cast structures of their unalloyed irons depending on the composition and the cooling rate. Figure 1.5 shows a representative cast structure of such irons.

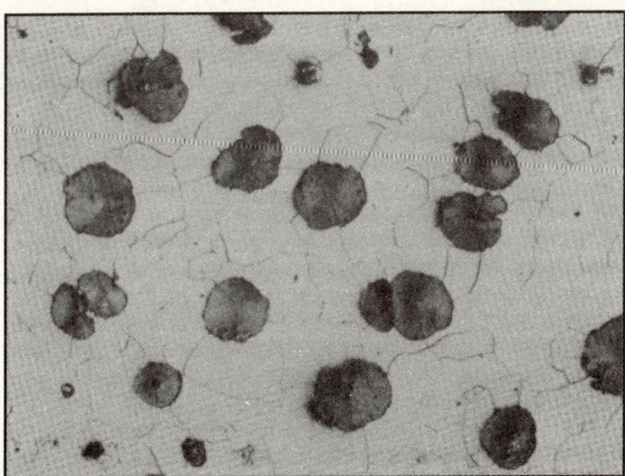

Fig. 1.5: S.G. cast iron showing nodules of graphite in matrix of ferrite, X150 (Courtesy of Portcullis Press, Redhill).

1.2.6 Vermicular Graphite (V.G.) Irons

These are the cast irons which are specially treated in the molten condition with small quantity of certain agents so as to cause precipitation of graphite in the cast structures having a shape which represents a transition (intermediate) form between flake and spheroidal graphite. From the points of view of compactness, the length to thickness ratio of such graphite is much smaller than the flake graphite but larger than the spheroidal graphite and therefore, such irons have properties intermediate between that of gray and spheroidal graphite irons in respect of the tensile strength and elongation. These irons are also called Compacted Graphite (CG) Irons. Figrue 1.6 shows a microstructure of CG iron.

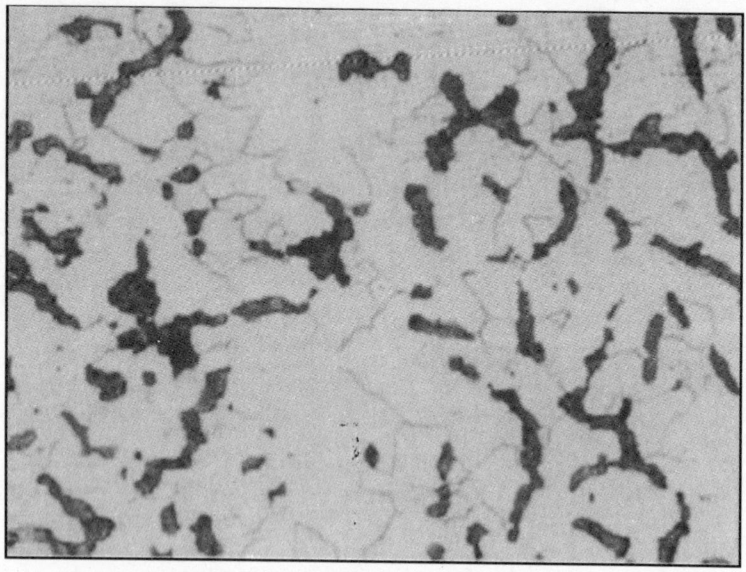

Fig. 1.6: Vermicular or compacted graphite iron showing graphite in matrix of ferrite, X100 (Reprinted with permission of ASM International).

1.3 CLASSIFICATION OF CAST IRONS

Cast irons have been classified in a number of ways using different basis by different authors. However, a more logical classification could be on the basis of the microstructure formed i.e. the form

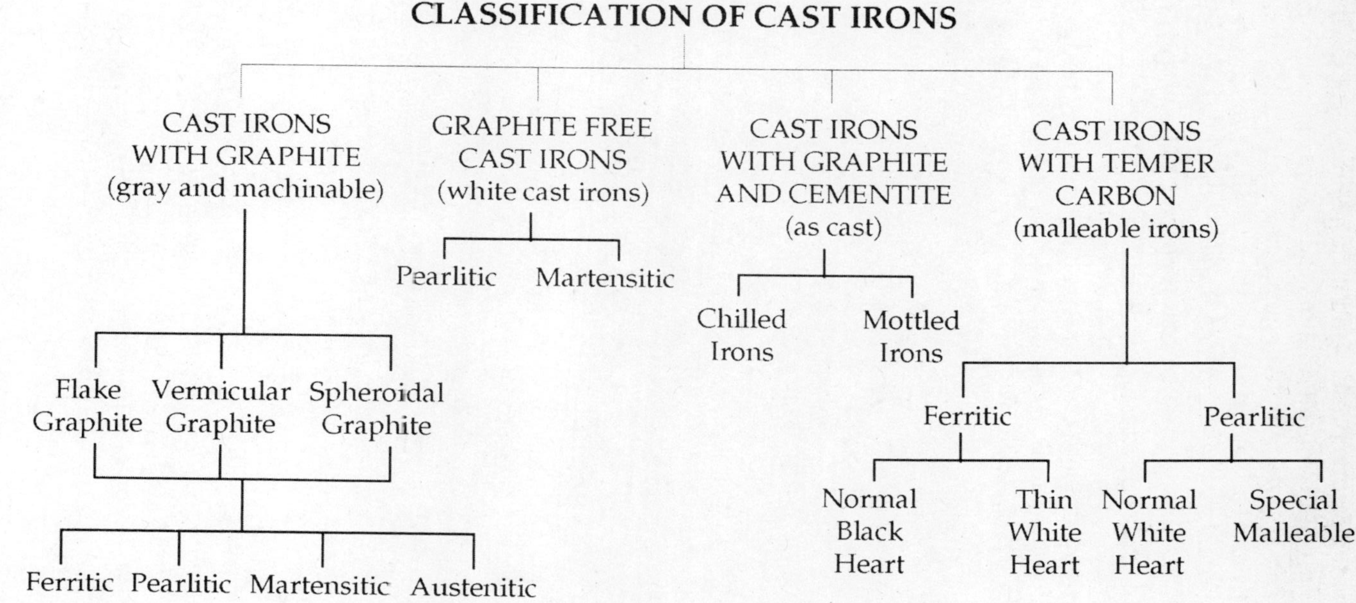
CLASSIFICATION OF CAST IRONS
CAST IRONS WITH GRAPHITE (gray and machinable)
GRAPHITE FREE CAST IRONS (white cast irons)
CAST IRONS WITH GRAPHITE AND CEMENTITE (as cast)
CAST IRONS WITH TEMPER CARBON (malleable irons)
Pearlitic
Martensitic
Chilled Irons
Mottled Irons
Flake Graphite
Vermicular Graphite
Spheroidal Graphite
Ferritic
Pearlitic
Normal Black Heart
Thin White Heart
Normal White Heart
Special Malleable
Ferritic
Pearlitic
Martensitic
Austenitic

and shape of the carbon present and the constituents of the matrix material. The use of commercial or trade name and application sometimes can also help in distinguishing the different categories of the cast irons available. As such, the classification of cast irons as shown in the form of a chart on page 7 can be suggested.

Hence, it is obvious that a variety of cast irons are available depending on their structures formed. They find different applications on the basis of their specific characteristics and properties. Some of these cast irons are also known by trade names which will be described while different groups of cast irons are discussed in the subsequent chapters.

Melting of Cast Irons

2.1 INTRODUCTION

Melting of cast iron is the process of producing liquid iron of the required composition at the required rate and with the required amount of melt superheat while incurring the minimum cost. It is a very important aspect of manufacture of iron castings as many defective castings may result from the incorrect composition and wrong melt superheat of iron supplied so much so that it may lead to total rejection of the casting. The proper selection and utilization of the melting units available therefore are of paramount importance for smooth, quality and economical production. A number of melting furnaces are available and understanding of characteristics of these furnaces such as the melting rate, fuel or energy requirement, charge materials to be melted, type of the labour required to operate and maintain, possibility of composition and temperature control etc. are necessary for the foundrymen before selecting a melting furnace.

2.2 TYPES OF MELTING FURNACES AND PRACTICE

Of all the foundry equipments used, the most important is a reliable melting unit capable of supplying consistent or regular quality of metal at the required superheat and at the right time or at the required rate. Many varieties of the cast iron melting units are available and can be classified in a number of ways such as depending on energy source used i.e. Fuel Fired and Electric Furnaces, on the basis of the tonnage handled and pattern of demand i.e. Batch Melting and Continuous Melting Furnaces. A more logical classification of these furnaces can be on the basis of their design and on this basis, various cast iron melting furnaces used in foundry can be divided into the following groups and subgroups:

1. Reverberatory Furnaces such as:
   (*i*) Fixed Air Furnaces
   (*ii*) Rotary Furnaces
2. Crucible Furnaces such as Coal fired, Oil fired or Gas fired Crucible Furnaces
3. Electric Furnaces such as
   (*i*) Induction Furnaces, both Coreless and Core type Furnaces
   (*ii*) Electric Arc Furnaces, both Direct Arc and Indirect Arc Furnaces
4. Shaft Furnaces such as Cupola and its various modifications

   These furnaces may be used either singly or incombination known as Duplexing or Duplex Melting (using two melting units). Under duplexing, various combinations of melting furnaces may be:

   (*i*) Cupola + Air Furnace
   (*ii*) Cupola + Rotary Furnace
   (*iii*) Cupola + Direct Arc Furnace
   (*iv*) Cupola + Either type Induction Furnace
   (*v*) Coreless Induction Furnace + Core type Induction Furnace

   The purpose of duplexing may be one or more of the following:

   (*i*) To provide a supply of hot metal so that the pouring can continue uninterrupted even if the primary melting unit or metal transfer facilities are out of order.
   (*ii*) To level out variations in metal temperature and composition from the primary melter.
   (*iii*) To adjust and/or maintain metal temperature and analysis within specified limits (i.e. superheating and/or refining the metal, as required).
   (*iv*) To maintain a supply of metal for continuous pouring when the primary melter is a batch type furnace such as electric furnace.
   (*v*) To accumulate sufficient metal to pour an unusually large size casting.

A very common purpose of duplexing is to control the composition and temperature of the iron produced. For example, a cupola may be used as a primary melter whereas, an air furnace or direct electric arc furnace may be used to reduce the carbon content and obtain the required melt superheat.

Each of the above melting units has its own special characteristics and limitations and is suitable for certain melting conditions. The design, melting practice, advantages and limitations and applications of each of the above melting units can be discussed as follows.

2.3 REVERBERATORY FURNACES

These furnaces are used when the molten cast irons with lower carbon content (<2.7%) and sulphur content (<0.08%) and with higher temperatures (>1450° C) are required. They are used mainly as primary melting unit for production of blackheart malleable irons, high duty and alloy cast irons with higher superheat and also for production of rolls requiring large amount of metal with precise chemical control. They are normally used on batch basis, but can be also used in duplex melting with cupolas where continuous melting and tapping is desired.

A reverberatory furnace in general, is a long, wide acid refractory lined furnace which is fired with fuel at one end and the heat produced is radiated and reflected down off the roof to the melting stock lying on the hearth. The exhaust gases exit at the opposing end to the burner. The charging is carried out through doors on the front of the furnace or through roof and the furnace is fired with oil, gas or pulverized coal. These furnaces use an extensive shallow metal bath and due to large slag-metal interfacial area available, an extensive refining with slag is possible. Silicon and manganese present in the iron are lost in the beginning during melting down period and the carbon is lost, later as temperature of the bath increases. The following reactions may take place:

$$\underline{Si} + O_2 = SiO_2$$

$$\underline{Si} + 2FeO = SiO_2 + 2Fe$$

$$\underline{Mn} + \frac{1}{2}O_2 = MnO$$

$$\underline{Mn} + FeO = MnO + Fe$$

$$\underline{C} + O_2 = CO_2$$
$$2\underline{C} + O_2 = CO$$

During melting down, the furnace gases such as O_2 and CO_2 may also form an iron oxide-rich skin on the iron and as the metal liquefies, silicon and manganese are oxidized by this iron oxide as shown in the above reactions. Losses due to such oxidation of silicon and manganese may be as high as 20% and carbon is lost upto 15%.

There are two types of reverberatory furnaces used for melting of cast irons:

1. Fixed Air Furnaces
2. Rotary Furnaces

2.3.1 Fixed Air Furnaces

Figure 2.1 shows a schematic sketch of a Fixed Air Furnace having an arched roof of fire bricks and the side walls which are lined with fire bricks and the bottom or hearth lined with silica or firebricks. The furnace is rectangular and may have inside width of 5 to 10 feet and length of 15 to 20 feet with melting capacity of 5 to 50 tons per heat (15 to 40 tons are most common). The furnace is tapped intermittently after a longer melting time of 4 to 12 hours and the pouring temperature varies from 1540 to 1600° C.

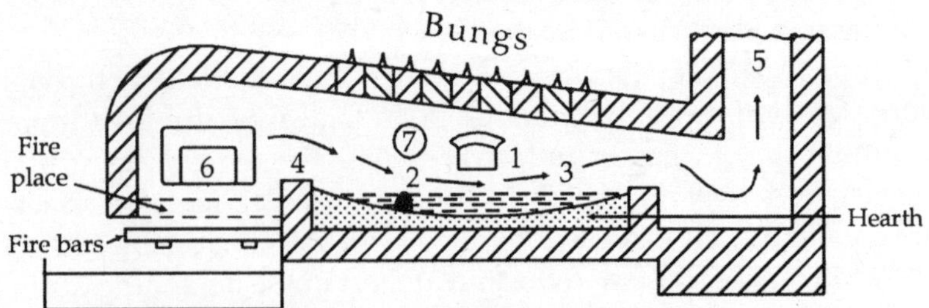

(1) Skimming door (2) Top hole (3) Molten iron (4) Fire bridge (5) Stack (6) Firing door (7) Sight hole

Fig. 2.1: Sectional View of an Air Furnace

Charging is done from the top of the roof by removing bungs which is replaced later on. The charge may consist of steel and cast iron scrap and pig iron. The sequence of charging is to put light scrap first on the hearth, followed by addition of malleable iron and steel scrap and finally the pig iron pieces so that the latter melts first and also protects smaller pieces from oxidation.

The use of such furnaces is now limited due to their lower thermal efficiency (~ 15%), larger melting time and higher fuel consumption. They also require high quality of fuel which is becoming expensive. The melting losses are also high, necessitating 30 to 40% of the pig iron in the charge which thus becomes a cost burden. Such furnaces are now being placed with rotary furnaces which are more flexible and thermally efficient.

2.3.2 Rotary Furnaces

These furnaces have cylindrical steel shell, with fire brick lining and are tapered and open at both ends (Fig. 2.2). They rotate at a slow speed of 1RPM and the continuous rotation starts only when the metal is molten. They use similar fuels as the air furnaces along with the preheated air and the melting conditions can be made neutral, oxidizing or reducing, as desired.

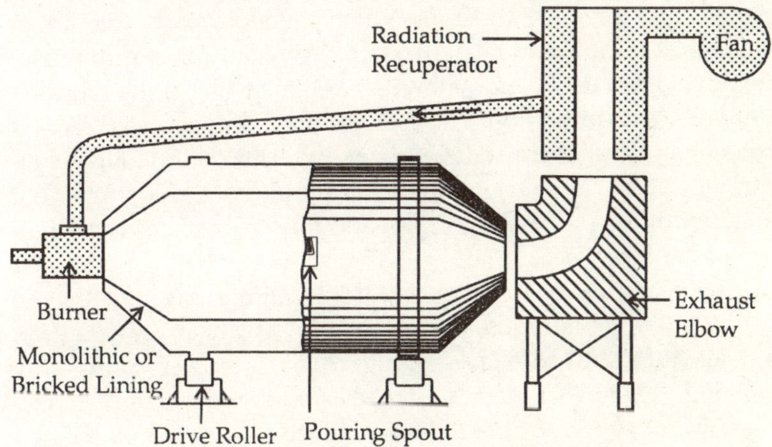

Fig. 2.2: Schematic Diagram of Rotary Furnace with Air Preheater (Reproduced with permission of Palgrave Macmillan).

These furnaces are more flexible than fixed air furnaces as any quantity of metal can be drawn at a time and the additions can be made in the furnace whenever desired by removing the exhaust box temporarily from the charging end.

Due to rotation of the furnace, the metal gets indirectly heated by conduction of heat from the walls in addition to receiving direct radiated heat from the flame and is thus melted more efficiently and faster. The melting time is reduced to almost half of that of the fixed furnace. The first heat may take 2 to 3 hours which is further reduced to $1\frac{1}{2}$ to 2 hours in the subsequent heats. As the furnace lining is heated, its heat is transferred to the underside of the metal charge during rotation and this overcomes the heat insulating effect of the slag formed.

The refractory lining has longer life and may be renewed after 200 to 300 heats. Due to preheated air supply, the flame temperature increases and the tapping temperature as high as 1600°C is obtained. The melting furnace may have capacity ranging from 1 to 50 tons preheat.

Rotary furnaces now find greater application than air furnace because of their above characteristics and are used for melting of high grade cast irons, malleable and ductile irons.

2.4 CRUCIBLE FURNACES

Crucible furnaces are those in which the stock to be melted is placed in a crucible and heated externally by oil, gas or pulverized coal or coke via heat conduction through the walls of the crucible. Therefore, contamination from the combustion products is not a problem and the melt produced is of excellent quality. However, the amount of the metal melted is limited by the low thermal efficiency of the process (3 to 18%) and thus a small batch melting is the usual practice.

Crucible furnaces used for cast iron melting may be either of lift-out or tilting type and have capacity varying from few hundred kg to less than one ton. Clay-graphite crucibles are very commonly used. Fig. 2.3 shows schematic sketches of a gas-fired and a coke-fired lift-out type crucible furnaces. Since the crucible is heated externally and there is no direct contact with the flame or products of the combustion, little oxidation and variation in the composition takes place. Further, as the melt produced is of smaller quantity, there is no problem in meeting the required degree of superheat.

Crucible furnaces are not very much in use for melting of cast irons due to their small capacities and the high cost of fuel used. However, such furnaces are employed to some extent when small quantity of molten metals of special composition such as white heart malleable iron or alloy cast iron are required.

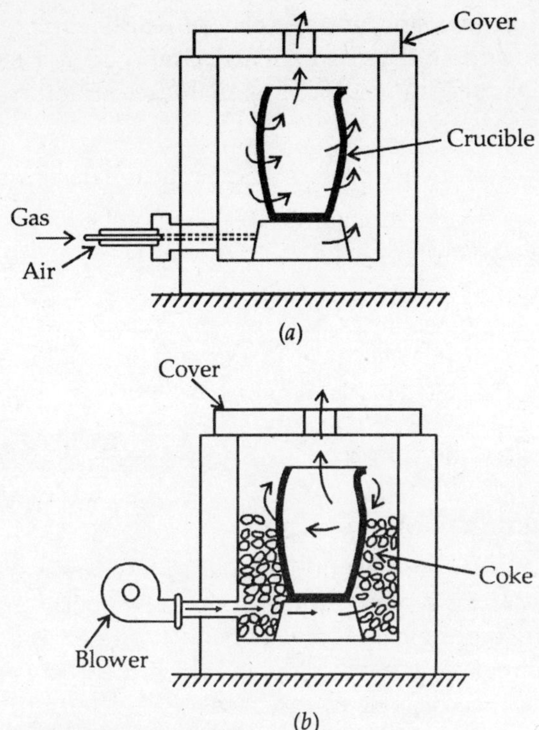

Fig. 2.3: Schematic Sketch of Crucible Furnaces (a) Gas-fired Crucible Furnace (*b*) Coke-fired Crucible Furnace

2.5 ELECTRIC FURNACES

The use of electric furnaces in which electrical power is used as a source of heat has increased considerably in recent years because of the cleaner and controlled melting. However, for melting of heavy pig iron and scrap used in cast iron melting, electric melting is much more expensive than other furnaces and its adoption depends upon availability of cheap electric power. However, there are a number of advantages which can serve to compensate for the extra cost incurred in electric melting. The advantages are :

(*i*) The composition of cast iron can be much more closely and precisely controlled, particularly the carbon content and the sulphur pick-up arising from use of fuels can be avoided.

(*ii*) There is reduction in the likelihood of metal contamination.

(*iii*) The metal can be superheated as required.

(*iv*) The turnings and borings can be readily utilized in their loose form as the charge material and do not require any special preparatory method such as briquetting to avoid oxidation losses

There are two major classes and their subclasses of electric furnaces:

1. Induction Furnaces
   (*i*) Coreless induction furnaces
   (*ii*) Core type induction furnaces
2. Arc Furnaces
   (*i*) Direct arc furnaces
   (*ii*) Indirect arc furnaces

2.5.1 Induction Furnaces

In these furnaces, no fuels or electrodes are used as a source of heat and the latter required for melting and superheating iron is produced in the metal itself; the metal bath being a complete secondary circuit of a transformer in which the heat is generated by the resistance offered to the passage of alternating current induced from the primary circuit of the transformer.

As mentioned above, there are two distinct types of induction furnaces:

1. Coreless or Channel Type Induction Furnace
2. Coreless Induction Furnace

Although, the above furnaces differ in construction appreciably, the principle of operation is same as described above.

2.5.1.1 Core Type or Channel Type Induction Furnaces

The construction of a channel type induction furnace is shown in Fig. 2.4. In this furnace, the primary coil is wound on a laminated iron core and around this core passes a channel containing the metal which is connected at its upper ends to the main bath of the furnace. The metal in the channel is heated and the electromagnetic forces cause a circulation between the channel and the main bath of the furnace. It is obvious that this type of furnace is difficult to start from cold as the channels must be first filled with metal.

Therefore, a precast plug of metal is used for starting from the cold and a heal of hot metal is left for the subsequent heats for next starting the furnace.

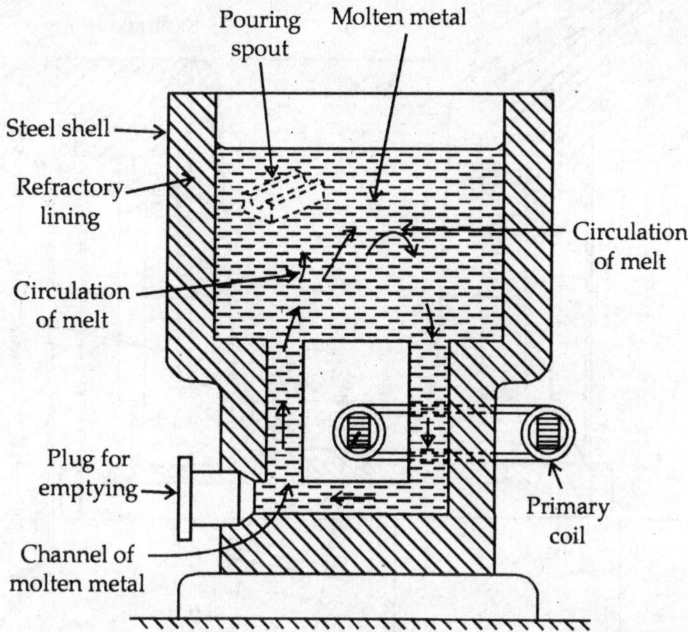

Fig. 2.4: Schematic Representation of a Channel Type Induction Furnace (Courtesy of Portcullis Press, Redhill).

The furnace operates on an a.c. supply of 50 or 60 cycles per second (i.e. on main or line current) and a typical melting unit having a capacity of 35 tons and power rating of 1500 KW will give a melting rate of 2500 kg per hour. Core type induction furnaces may have capacities as large as 270 tons. Such furnaces are efficient melter, the thermal efficiency being about 80%. They are, however, best suited for holding and superheating work.

2.5.1.2 Core Less Induction Furnaces

Such induction furnaces consist of a refractory crucible (of silica or magnesite) placed centrally (Fig. 2.5) inside a water-cooled copper coil and packed into position by ramming dry insulatory refractory between the crucible and the copper coil. They can be tilting type or lift-coil type. They are simpler in construction as compared to core-type but have lower thermal efficiency (upto 60%) as compared to core type.

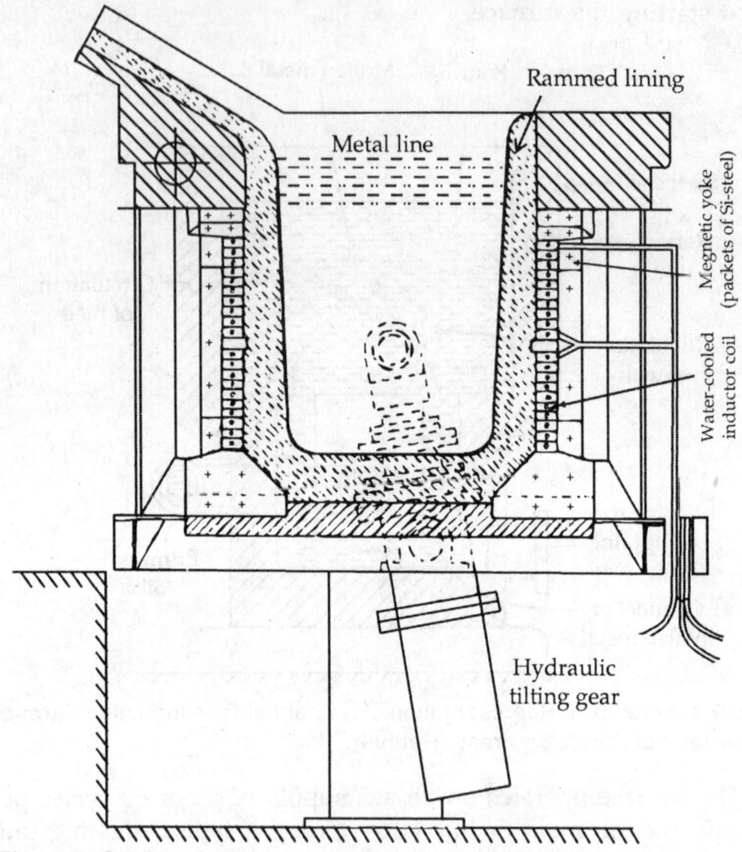

Fig. 2.5: Schematic Representation of a Coreless Induction Furnace (Courtesy of Portcullis Press, Redhill).

There are two types of coreless induction furnaces :

(*i*) High or Medium Frequency Furnaces operating on 500 to 10,000 cycles per second.

(*ii*) Mains Frequency Furnaces operating on mains frequency i.e. 50 or 60 cycles per second.

Both of the above types of induction furnaces are similar in construction. High frequency furnaces easily melt small pieces of cold metal (cast iron borings) and they are used in preference to the mains frequency furnaces for rapid melting of small heats and when operations require frequent changes in the composition of the metal to be melted and poured and hence, more flexible. However, high frequency furnaces require expensive motor generator set-up and therefore, their capacities are limited to about 12 tons. They also find limited application in cast iron melting due to their high capital costs associated with the requirement of motor generator set-up.

The mains frequency coreless induction furnaces have been recently developed which eliminate the need of expensive motor generator or converter. The operation and maintenance of such furnaces are simpler and the stirring action is greater in such furnaces as compared to high frequency ones ensuring a complete homogenization of the melt. This is because the stirring effect varies inversely with the square root of the frequency. But mains frequency furnaces, like core type furnaces, require a heal of molten metal to be left in the furnace after tapping to form the secondary circuit. This metal may amount to some 25 to 30% of the total capacity of the furnace. This fact rather limits their use when frequent changes in compositions are required in the charges being melted and as such, they must be used on a continuous melting basis. Typical capacities of such furnaces may vary from less than one ton to 40 tons with as large power rating of as 7000 kW. There are furnaces which have melting rate of over 100 tons per hour.

In general, induction melting practice may be on batch basis or continuous basis, the latter accounting for most of the tonnage melted. These furnaces have advantages in that

(*i*) No metal contamination by electrodes or fuels
(*ii*) A homogeneous melt is obtained and melting losses are minimum
(*iii*) Any degree of superheat can be obtained.

The charges in induction melting furnaces for grey cast iron melting are usually made of steel and cast iron scraps, foundry returns, ferrosilicon and carbon in suitable proportions to provide the desirable composition of the iron. Pig iron is seldom used. A typical charge composition may consist of 41.3% steel scrap, 10% grey iron borings, 45% foundry returns, 1.7% carbon and 2% FeSi.

Like reverberatory furnaces, iron melted in induction furnaces passes through a melting down stage in the beginning of the heat and silicon and manganese are lost by oxidation reactions as described in the case of above furnaces. The melting conditions are acid as the both furnace lining used as well as slag formed are acid. As the temperature increases, silica reduction by carbon in the metal becomes important and the following reaction may take place at high temperature:

$$SiO_2 + 2\underline{C} = \underline{Si} + 2CO$$

This leads to silicon pick up in the iron. For this, silica is available both from slag and refractory lining. Molten cast irons also may decarburize rapidly at high temperatures when the furnace atmosphere is made of air, and/or CO_2. The following reactions may take place:

$$\underline{C} + O_2 = CO_2$$

or

$$2\underline{C} + O_2 = 2CO$$

At high temperature when carbon is capable of reducing oxides like silica, no slag scum forms and the melt surface becomes clear.

Coreless induction furnaces are used as primary melter on both batch basis and continuous basis. The latter is, however, the major use of induction melting. The general practice is to use several mains frequency induction furnaces together and tapping 10 to 30% of the capacity of each furnace in rotation and immediately adding to them the same amount of the fresh charge. In this way, transfer or pour ladles are kept full in pace with the production line. A holding channel type induction furnace is not necessary but its presence will add to the flexibility of the process. Induction furnaces of both the coreless and core type are also used in duplex melting operations.

2.5.2 Electric Arc Furnaces

In electric arc furnaces, the heat required for melting and superheating the metal is supplied by electric arc struck between the electrodes and/or the metal and the temperature of the arc exceed 3000° C. The melting is very rapid and control over temperature and composition of metal produced is excellent. The melting stock commonly used consists of solid pieces of pig iron, steel and cast iron scrap and foundry returns along with addition of carburizers and ferroalloys, as may be required. Two types of electric arc furnaces are used:

1. Direct Arc Furnace
2. Indirect Arc Furnace

2.5.2.1 *Direct Arc Furnace*

Such furnaces are also known as Arc-Resistance Furnaces as the heat is provided by the radiation from an arc formed between the electrodes and the melting charge as well as to a lesser extent by the resistance of the charge to the passage of the current. A 3-phase power supply is used and one phase is connected to each of the 3 electrodes used. The arc is regulated by automatic controls, which raise or lower the electrodes to maintain the desired arc voltage. Electrodes arc of graphite or amorphous carbon. The current is supplied through a transformer which permits voltage to be varied according to the stage of the process and heavy input required.

All the direct arc furnaces used are of tilting type, provided with a bowl shaped hearth and dome shaped roof (Fig. 2.6) which may be removable by sliding or swinging. The charging may be from the top of the roof by bucket either by removing the roof by swinging or sliding. The furnace may be also chute-charged through a side charging door. The lining of the various parts of the furnace arc different due to different service requirements. The bottom being generally basic (using rammed dolomite mixture or magnesite mix) and the side walls are made of high alumina fire bricks. The roof is usually made of silica bricks, although nowadays, they are being replaced by high alumina fire bricks.

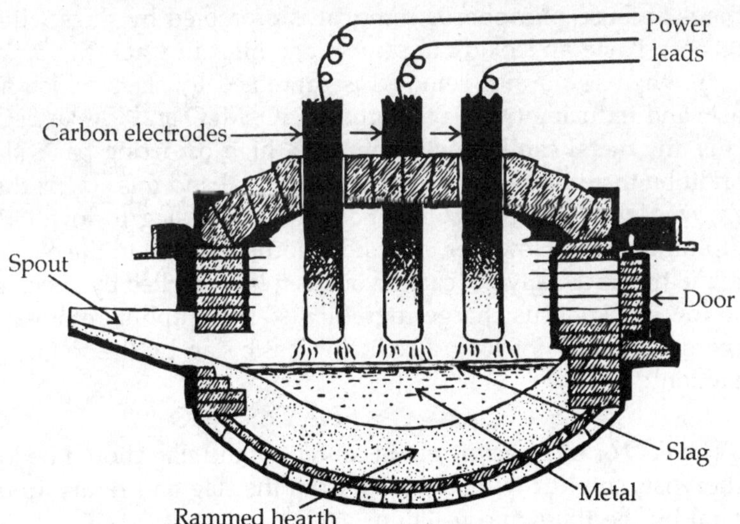

Fig. 2.6: Schematic Sketch of Direct Arc Furnace

The direct arc furnace can be successfully employed for different types of metal charges. The latter can be either the normal mixture of pig iron and scrap or those containing upto 100% of steel scrap when necessary carburization of the metal can be effected by the addition of crushed graphite electrodes or some other suitable material like coke breeze etc. and the ferro alloys can be added for the production of alloy cast irons. The furnace can melt any size of the charge material consisting of 100% borings to heavy structural steel scrap.

The furnace capacity can range from 1 to 100 tons, most common being 2 to10 tons. The average power consumption for melting a cold charge is 500 KWh/ton of iron. To save power consumption and increase the production rates by over 30%, there are several installations in operation where the charges used are preheated. As mentioned earlier, the power applied varies according to the stage of melting and refining. Full power is applied during melting down requiring high heat input and during refining a lower voltage is used. For a 8 tons heat, the voltage applied may be varied in 4 stages as 240, 165, 125 and 95 volts at a current of 8000 Amp. The melting time of a furnace heat may vary from $1\frac{1}{2}$ to 2 hours from tap to tap for a batch melting operation.

Removal of sulphur and phosphorus is possible in direct arc furnace melting conditions using "double-slag" making operations. This is because phosphorus removal is promoted by slags which are both basic and oxidizing (i.e. slags high in CaO, MgO and FeO), whereas sulphur removal is promoted by slags which are basic and reducing (i.e. slags high in CaO, MgO and low in FeO). Thus, the metal can be melted under a high oxidizing basic slag condition to accomplish phosphorus removal and this slag is then removed and replaced with a basic reducing slag to lower the sulphur content. However, the phosphorus removal in the electric arc melting is usually not carried out as it is controlled by choosing the low-phosphorus charge ingredients. The sulphur removal is accomplished by forming a reducing basic slag by the following reaction :

$$\underline{S} + CaO + C = Fe + CaS + CO$$

The FeO or other acidic oxide content of the slag should be low otherwise, sulphur will pass back from the slag and return to the metal by the following reaction:

$$CaS + 2FeO = CaO + FeO + \underline{S}$$

2.5.2.1.1 *Advantages of Direct Arc Furnace*

In general, the advantages of direct electric arc melting are:

(*i*) It permits complete flexibility in type of slag maintained, range of raw materials usable and type of products made (i.e. all grades of iron can be prepared). Arc furnace can melt any kind of scrap from 100% borings to heavy structural steels.
(*ii*) The melting efficiency is very high ~ 80%.

2.5.2.1.2 *Limitations of Direct Arc Furnace*

The main limitations of direct arc melting are:

(*i*) Its high capital cost per unit of output
(*ii*) The electrode consumption is considerable item in operating costs
(*iii*) The melting operation is noisy
(*iv*) There is a severe overheating of the melt under the electrodes thus, impairing the quality of the product.

The direct arc furnaces are most commonly employed either as batch melting unit or as a holding, superheating and refining furnace in conjunction with cupola in duplex melting practice.

2.5.2.2 *Indirect Arc Furnace*

These furnaces (also known as Arc-Radiation Furnaces) are used mainly for melting of small quantities of special cast irons like alloy cast irons. The indirect arc furnace is a barrel shaped furnace (Fig. 2.7) mounted on rollers and rotated to-and-fro during melting to rock continuously and thus permitting intimate contact between the lining and the charge and thereby promoting heat transfer to the charge and prolonging the life of the furnace acid lining. Thus the metal is heated indirectly through this mode of heat transfer by conduction as well as directly by radiation from the arc struck between the electrodes.

Two carbon electrodes are used for striking the arc and a single phase power supply is employed. The size of these furnaces are thus limited to less than one ton by the necessity of avoiding too large a single phase load. For charging through an end, the electrodes are removed and repositioned once the charge has subsided. Charging is also done sometimes through an opening provided for the same. Pouring spout is also built with the charging door.

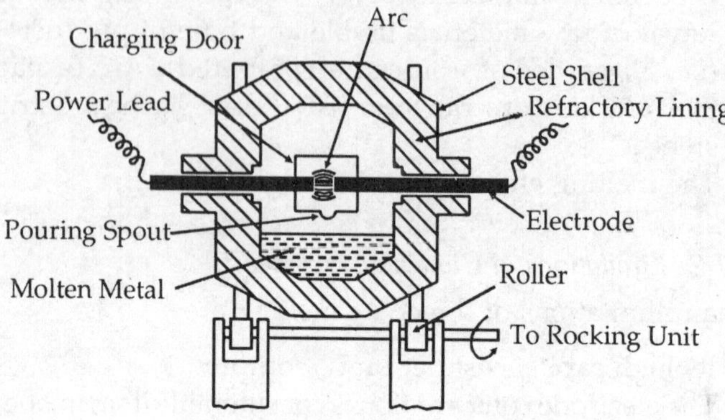

Fig. 2.7: Schematic Sketch of Indirect Arc Furnace

Indirect arc furnaces have much the same advantages as the direct arc. However, due to their small size and noisy operation, they are used to a minor extent in cast iron foundry industry. They are also not so versatile in slag practice as the direct arc furnace, although the local over heating of the charge is comparatively much less in such furnaces.

2.6 SHAFT FURNACES

Cupola and its various modifications are the examples of shaft melting furnaces which are most commonly used for cast iron produced and about 90% of cast irons produced are melted in cupola, particularly the gray irons and alloy cast irons. The development of the blast furnace gave birth to cupola melting. Earlier, the pig iron produced in blast furnace was directly used for making iron castings. As the time went on, smaller shaft-type furnaces were designed for remelting of solid pig iron and scrap materials for making gray iron castings.

2.6.1 Conventional Cupola

The conventional cupolas are acid-lined and use cold air blast for combustion of the fuel. A cupola is a vertical shaft furnace (Fig. 2.8) into which is placed the metal to be melted, a flux like

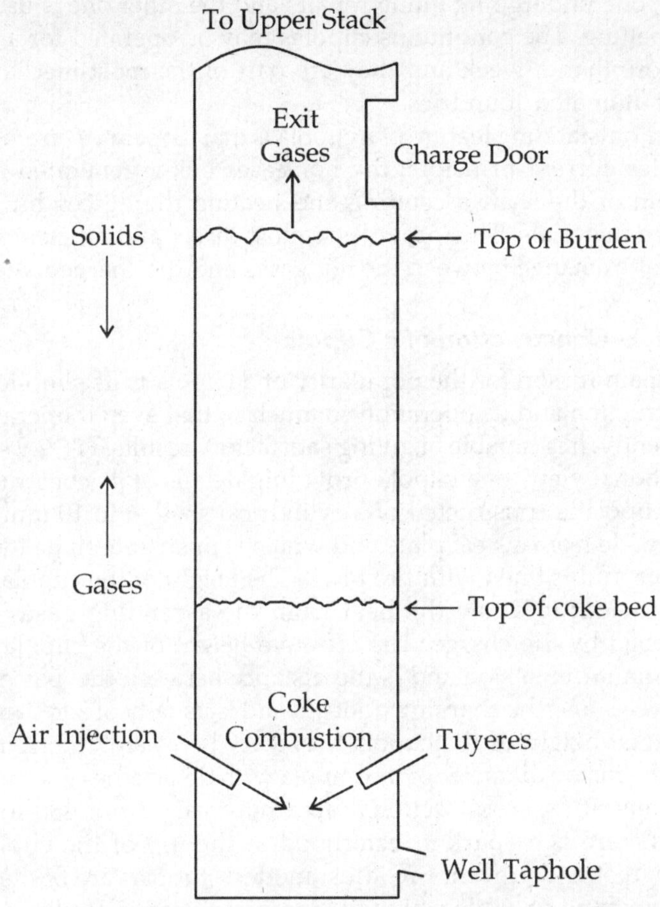

Fig. 2.8: Basic Components of a Cupola Melting Furnace

limestone for slag forming and a fuel like coke which is burnt by air being passed through tuyeres. It is equipped with a wind box and tuyeres for admitting air, a charging door at the top for admitting charge materials, a tap hole and a slag hole in intermittent type small cupolas for removal of metal and slag and a sand bottom at the base. Most medium and large size cupolas, however, operate on continuous basis i.e. metal and slag flows through the same door continuously and are separated in a basin in the spout outside the cupola with the help of a slag dam. The small cupolas which are operated on a batch basis are used in pairs, one undergoing lining repairs and the other one is used for the melting. The continuous cupolas may be operated for a week or more than a week and they are part of the most mechanized and automated foundries.

The outstanding feature of a cupola is that it operates on a unique counter current principle: the hot gases being generated at the bottom of the shaft ascending and heating the descending cold charge materials. This provides a most direct and efficient mode of heat exchange between the hot gases and the charge materials.

2.6.1.1 Construction of a Cupola

The main reason for the popularity of a cupola is its simplicity of construction and its operation so much so that even if operated in efficiently, it is capable of giving satisfactory results. Fig. 2.9 shows a sectional view of a cupola providing details of its construction. The cupola is constructed of a cylindrical shell, 6 to 10 mm thick and made from a steel plate and which is open at both its top and bottom and is lined with fire brick. The height of the cupola shaft is sufficient to allow the heat from the ascending gases to be absorbed by the charge. The effective height of the cupola is an important dimension and is the distance between the axis of row of tuyeres and the charging door sill and is usually of 5 to 7 metres. The total height of the cupola may vary between 7 to 12 metres and the inside diameter of the cupola with determines the capacity and operating cross sectional area may vary from 450 to 2500 mm. There is a spark arresterhood at the top of the cupola to catch dust and prevent fire. Most modern cupolas are of the drop bottom type in which hinged doors are placed under a sand bottom, allowing the bottom to be lowered at the end of the cupola heat to aid cleaning.

The air from the blower comes through a blast pipe and enters the wind box which surrounds the cupola and supplies air evenly to all the tuyeres which are equally spaced around the circumference of the cupola and blow equal quantities of air for uniform combustion in the coke bed. The total cross sectional area of all the tuyers is usually 1/4 or 1/8th of the internal cross sectional area of the cupola at the tuyer level. The number of tuyers required increases with increase in cupola diameter and may usually vary between 4 to 10. The cupola is generally rated in its capacity by its inside diameter. The output rate of the cupola is designated in terms of its melting rate which varies in the range of 1 to 50 tons per hour and may be as large as even 100 tons per hour.

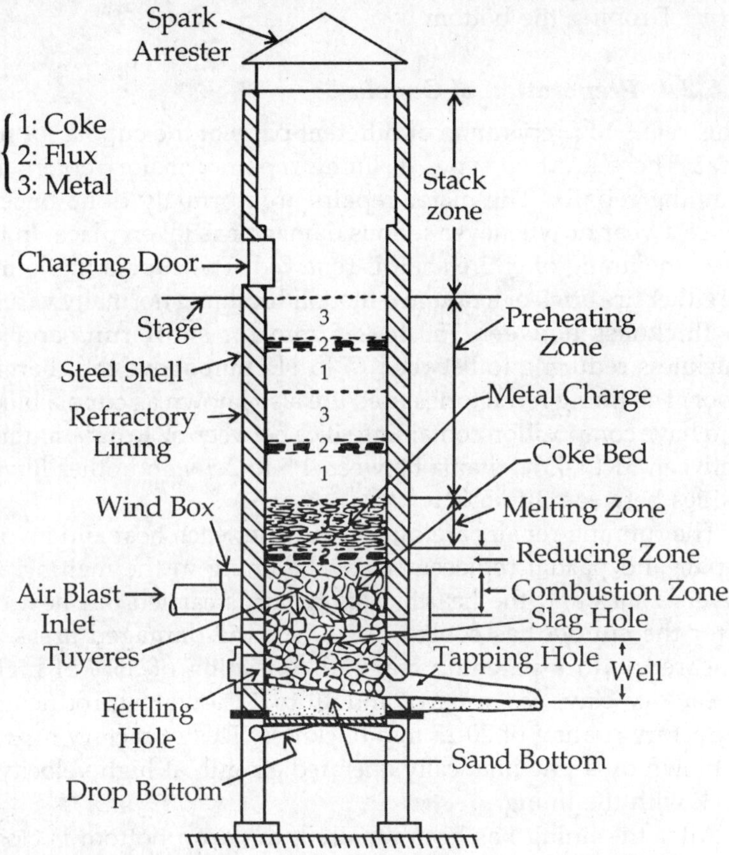

Fig. 2.9: Sectional View of a Conventional Cupola Providing Details of Its Construction

2.6.2 Operation of Cupola

For a successful cupola heat, a number of melting operations are required which occur each time a heat is made. The various steps involved in cupola operation are:

(*i*) Preparation of cupola (including preparation and repair of lining, bottom, tap and slag holes)

(*ii*) Lighting the fire in the coke bed (also known as burning or putting in the coke bed)

(*iii*) Charging
(*iv*) Melting
(*v*) Slagging and Tapping
(*vi*) Droping the bottom

2.6.2.1 Preparation of Cupola

This refers to preparation of different parts of the cupola for next heat. There are two types of lining repairs : major repairs and running repairs. The major repairs are normally done once or twice a year or whenever serious damage has taken place. In this case, the lining of entire shaft is renewed. The cupola lining may be either fire brick or a rammed monolithic lining normally varying in thickness between 150 to 225 mm for short runs and the thickness reducing to between 75 to 112 mm above the charging door. The lining refractories used are also known as cupola blocks and have composition containing silica between 52 to 62%, alumina between 31 to 43%, titania between 1.5 to 2.5% and other fluxing oxides between 3 to 6%.

The running repairs are carried out after each heat and involve repair and partial replacement of the lining in the melting and tuyers zones and the hearth. This repair is carried out next day after the cupola has cooled down. All the damaged areas are smeared with a patching material consisting of 35% of highly refractory clay, 65% quartz and 10 to 12% water producing a refractory coating of 20-25 mm thickness. This refractory mixture is blown by a pneumatically operated air gun at high velocity to stick with the lining.

After the lining has been repaired, the drop bottom is closed and the bottom of the cupola is prepared by ramming a tempered moulding sand having 3 to 6% moisture and 60 or more permeability and sloping towards the tap hole for easy flow of molten metal.

2.6.2.2 Lighting the Fire in the Coke Bed

The cupola is kindled, one to two hours before the melting begins. An even layer of dry wooden chips is spread over the bottom and then some coke is added. The working door is then sealed with a brick and the wood is ignited through a hole left in the working door. When the coke is burning well, more coke is added and the hot burning coke pile is build up to a prescribed height to constitute what is known as 'Coke-Bed Height'. This is a critical height of the column of coke bed above the tuyers before charging begins. This height depends on the quality of the coke used and the volume and pressure of the blast blown. A correct bed height (usually 50 to 125 cm) is necessary for satisfactory working of the cupola and is ensured by measured it with the help of a chain or rod by lowering it from the charging door sill down to the top of the coke bed. Air, at about half the normal blowing rate is blown through this coke bed for 2 to 3 minutes to raise the coke temperature to a white heat, before charging begins.

2.6.2.3 Charging

Charging consists of adding weighed quantities of metal, coke and flux from the charging door. A small quantity of flux is first charged onto the coke bed followed by alternating layers of metal, coke and flux upto the lower sill of the charging door. The ratio of metallic charge to coke by weight varies depending on the compositions of metal and fuel used and ranges in various practices from about 4:1 to 12:1.The size of various charge ingredients used varies from practice to practice. Usually the size of coke and flux pieces are of the order of 40 to 50 mm. The amount of coke required varies depending upon several factors like coke quality, composition and size of metal charges etc. The flux charge usually varies from 2 to 4% by weight of the metal charge.

2.6.2.4 Melting

After the charging is complete, the charge materials are heated up with natural draught for 30 minutes to one hour. The slag and tap holes are closed using a conical clay plug and then the blowers are started for a few minutes. After about 10 minutes, molten iron starts accumulating in the hearth. The droplets of molten iron can be seen falling past the tuyeres through pee-holes. The molten iron along with slag formed is allowed to collect for about five minutes before tapping and slagging take place in a sequence.

2.6.2.5 Slagging and Tapping

After enough molten metal has been collected, the slag hole is opened, collected in a container and disposed off. In small cupolas, intermittent tapping requires that the tap hole be opened at intervals to deliver the iron to pouring ladles. For tapping, the tap hole is pierced using a short tapping bar. After the required quantity of the metal has been tapped or as soon as slag appears, the tap hole is sealed with a clay plug which is in the form of a small cone fitted on a steel disk of the bolt stick. The intervals of the tapping are predictable since the capacity of the ladles and melting rate of a cupola are known. Normally, the first iron can be tapped 35 to 45 minutes after the blast has commenced. Ordinarily, a slag hole is first opened about 30 to 45 minutes after the blast is on in order to allow time for sufficient slag to accumulate.

In large cupolas, where continuous tapping of iron is commonly done, use of some type of a dam on the spout is made. Such an arrangement is shown in Fig. 2.10. Critical dimensions in this system are the heights of the metal and slag dams above the top of the tap hole.

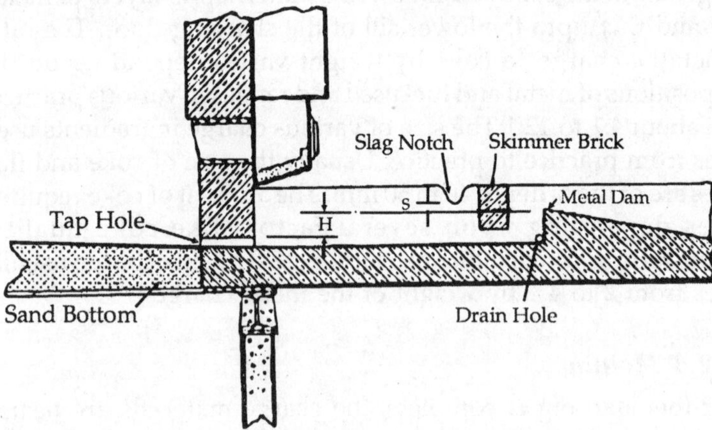

Fig. 2.10: Cross-section of a Continuous Tapping Spout (From AFS The Cupola and its Operation, 3rd edn., 1965).

2.6.2.6 Dropping the Bottom

At the end of a cupola heat, the charging is stopped and all the contents of the charge are allowed to melt till one or two charges are left above the coke bed. At this stage, the air blast is reduced and then stopped. The prop under the bottom door is knocked down and the contents of the cupola fall onto the floor under the cupola. Water is sprayed over such materials and the metal and coke are recovered from the same for use in the next heat.

2.6.3 Cupola Charge Materials

The cupola charge will consist of metallic materials, fuel and flux. The metallic portion of the charge includes pig iron, steel and cast iron scrap, foundry returns and ferro alloys. The selection of the above constituents must be carefully done. The fuel employed is the coke and the limestone ($CaCO_3$) along with other materials such as fluorspar (CaF_2), sodium carbonate (Na_2CO_3) etc. are the flux used for forming the slag.

The Pig Iron (PI): The pig iron used is a foundry grade PI (a blast furnace product) which is high in C, Si and Mn and sometimes in phosphorus as well. The composition of such iron could be 3.25 to 4% C, 1.25 to 4% Si, 0.25 to 1.25% Mn, 0.02 to 1.50% P.

The Scrap: This may include gray iron, malleable iron and steel scrap obtained from the production units as well as the market. Such scrap should be preferably free from certain undesirable elements like Sb, Sn, Pb, Zn, Al etc. which can be harmful to the iron produced.

The Foundry Return: This may include parts of the sprue, gates, risers and defective castings.

The proper proportioning of the above metallic charge constituents is performed by calculation for a particular composition of the iron to be produced. A typical composition of metallic charge ingredients may be 30% PI, 30% scrap and 40% foundry return.

In addition to above metallic charge materials, a number of alloying agents are utilized in the cupola charge in the form of additions like FeSi, FeMn, silicon carbide etc.

Coke: A foundry coke is produced from bituminous coals in by-product or beehive coke ovens, the by-product is in more general use. It is necessary that the foundry coke does not burn so readily as blast furnace coke. It is therefore generally carbonized for longer times. The coke should be low in ash and sulphur and should have good mechanical strength. The recommended composition of such coke is that it should have moisture 3% maximum, volatile matter, 2% maximum, fixed carbon, 86% minimum, ash, 12% maximum and 1% maximum sulphur.

Fluxes: These are the materials which react with the coke ash and melted refractory to make a fluid slag. Most commonly used fluxing agents are limestone, fluorspar and soda ash. The limestone used should have low acid oxide content and about 98% pure. Some of the limestone are replaced by dolomitic limestone having 15 to 30% $MgCO_3$.

2.6.4 The Cupola Melting Process

The cupola is designed not only for melting of cast iron but also for heating it to a temperature to provide sufficient fluidity to the metal. Cupola is essentially a melting unit and not a refining unit, although some changes in composition of the metal do take place due to presence of oxidizing gases and absorption of carbon and sulphur from the coke. Fig. 2.11 shows the basic reactions which occur during cupola melting process. Thus, the gases in cupola at various levels essentially consist of CO_2, CO, O_2 and N_2 with varying amounts of H_2O and H_2 depending upon the humidity of the air blast.

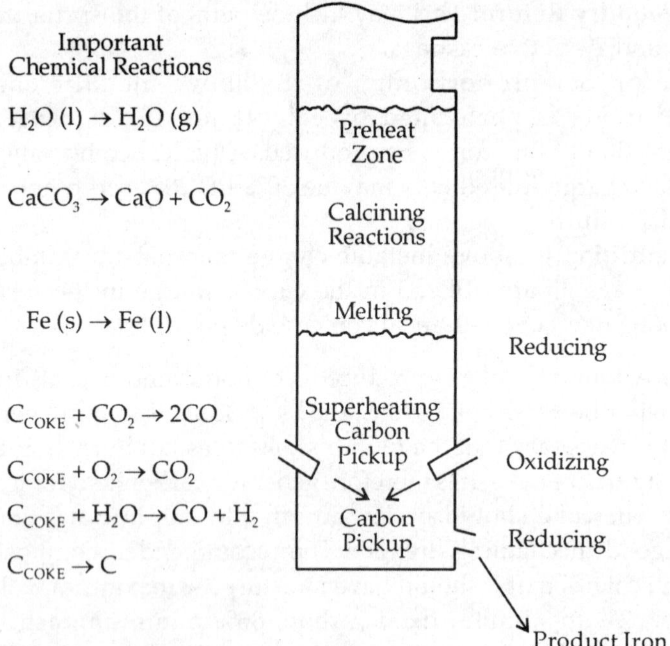

Fig. 2.11: Basic Reactions in the Cupola Melting Process

2.6.4.1 *Cupola Zones and Gases*

According to the temperature and composition of the gases present, the cupola may be divided into five basic zones which are shown diagrammatically in Fig. 2.12. The shape of these zones may vary depending upon several factors and the different reactions which may occur in these zones are explained as follows.

(*i*) **The Hearth or Crucible Zone:** This is the portion located between the lower edge of the tuyeres and the bottom of the cupola. In this zone, no combustion takes place. Under normal conditions, the gases in this zone are in equilibrium with the carbon of the coke and consist exclusively of CO. The hearth is filled with incandescent coke and a part of the carbon of the coke is transferred to the iron.

(*ii*) **The Oxidizing or Combustion Zone:** It is located above the hearth and it is here that intensive combustion (oxidation) of the coke takes place by the oxygen of the blast. The gases are highly oxidizing. In this zone, the oxidation of Si and Mn also occurs and this is accompanied by the liberation of an additional heat which superheats the molten droplets of the iron trickling into the hearth. Various reactions which take place in this zone are:

$$C + O_2 = CO_2 + \text{Heat}$$

The above reaction may take place in two steps as under:

$$C + \frac{1}{2}O_2 = CO + \text{Heat}$$

$$CO + \frac{1}{2}O_2 = CO_2$$

Other reaction are:

$$\underline{Si} + O_2 = SiO_2 + \text{Heat}$$

$$\underline{Mn} + \frac{1}{2}O_2 = MnO + \text{Heat}$$

The physical limits of this zone are the points of entry of air and the level where the free oxygen concentration in the gas is reduced to one per cent or less.

(*iii*) **The Reducing Zone:** This zone is located above the combustion zone and extends upto the top of the coke bed. In this zone, the reduction of CO_2 to CO occurs and the

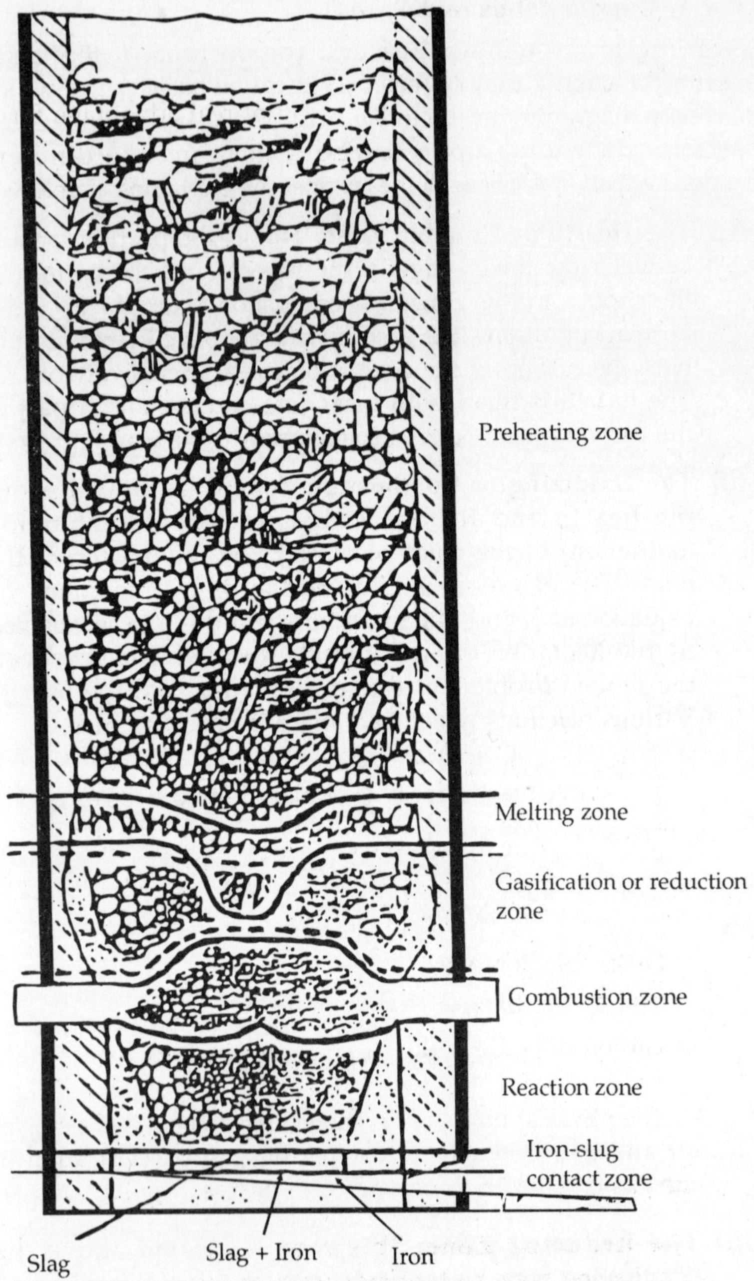

Fig. 2.12: Schematic Representation of Various Cupola Zones

temperature of the gases drops from 1600° C (in the combustion zone) to 1200° C at the coke bed. Due to reducing atmosphere, the charge is well protected from the oxidizing influence. The following reaction takes place :

$$CO_2 + C = 2CO - \text{Heat}$$

(*iv*) **The Melting Zone:** This refers to the layer of the molten iron just above the coke bed. The charge starts melting here and the molten iron trickles down through the coke bed to the bottom of the cupola. A considerable carbon pick-up by the molten iron may also occur in this zone according to the reaction:

$$2Fe + 2CO = Fe_3C + CO_2$$

(*v*) **Preheating Zone:** This zone occupies the space between the upper limit of the melting zone to the charging door. In this zone, moisture is evaporated and the volatile matter is, removed and the charge materials are heated up. The limestone is burnt and dissociates at about 700°C according to the reaction:

$$CaCO_3 = CaO + CO_2$$

In this zone, CO_2 and CO contents of the gases remain almost unchanged but the temperature of the gases fall due to heat absorption by the charge.

It has been found that the normal ratio of CO_2 to CO in cupola gases is approximately 2 to 1, two-thirds of the carbon being burned to form carbon-di-oxide and one-third forming carbon mono-oxide. The content of the products of combustion of carbon and oxygen in the cupola gases at various levels in the cupola shaft from the tuyeres to the charging door is shown in Fig. 2.13. The maximum amount of carbon-di-oxide and oxygen is observed at about 30 cm above the plane of the bottom row of tuyeres. As the amount of oxygen decreases, CO_2 content rapidly drops to about 15% and there is practically no change upto the level of charging door. The CO content increases upto the cupola shaft until a level of about 60 cm above the plane of the tuyeres is reached after which it is almost steady at about 9%.

Fig. 2.14 illustrates the change in the temperature of the gases as they rise up the cupola shaft. Thus the curves in above two figures show that the maximum CO_2 content corresponds to the highest gas temperature producing superheating zone in the cupola. As the CO_2 content decreases and the CO content increases the temperature of the cupola gases falls. A further drop in shaft gas temperature with the constant CO_2 and CO content is caused by the heat removal from the gases for heating up the charge materials moving downward.

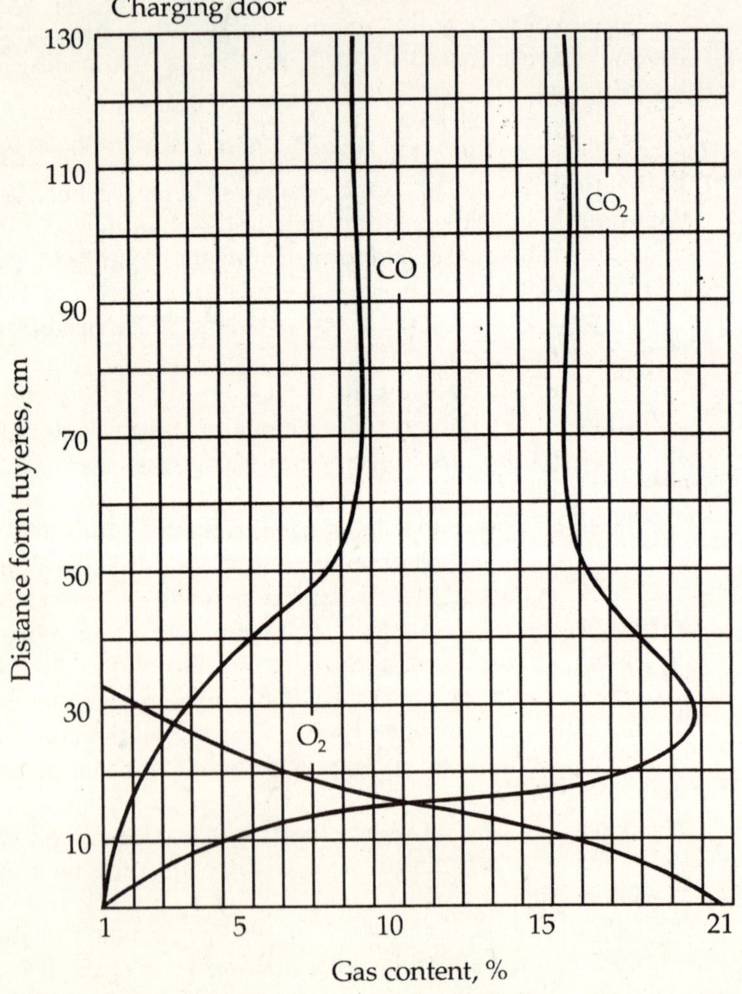

Fig. 2.13: Variation in Gas Content up Cupola Shaft for a Typical Cupola Size

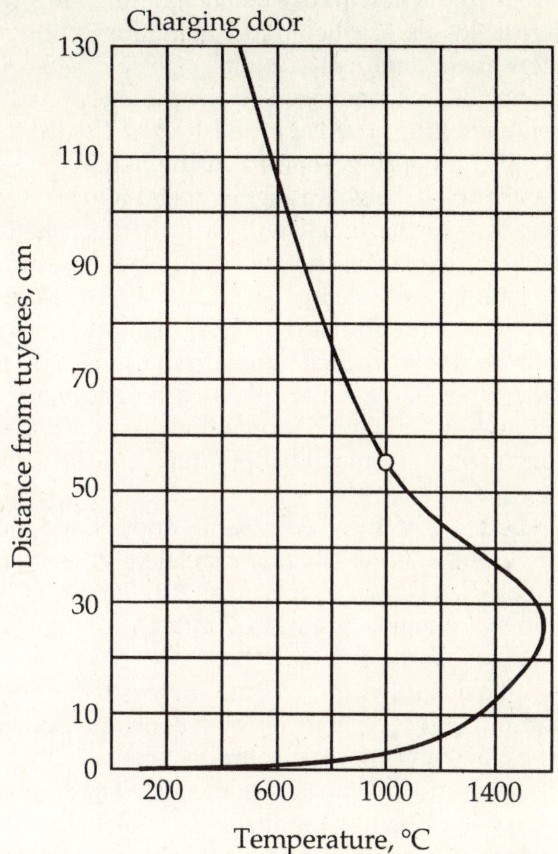

Fig. 2.14: Variation in Gas Temperature up Cupola Shaft

2.6.5 Control of Cupola Melting

The rate at which coke is charged in cupola and the air supply is made must be properly balanced. Maintenance of a proper coke bed height is also of paramount importance. Assuming that a proper coke bed height is maintained, the balance between coke and air supply can be judged from the composition of the stack gases. When the two of the above items are in unbalanced supply, certain metallurgical problems will arise. An excess of coke results in wastage of coke, a slow melting rate, a high percentage of carbon in the iron, lower metal temperature, excessive refractory erosion and other operation difficulties. On the other hand, an over-supply of air causes the reduction in coke bed height resulting in oxidation of iron, higher losses of silicon and manganese, low carbon in iron, and low metal temperature.

Maintenance of a proper coke bed height is reflected in several ways. During melting, the coke bed height fluctuates as coke descends into the melting zone from the stack above it. If the coke bed is at proper height, a higher metal temperature results. The temperature of the metal will drop if the coke bed burns away because of excess in the air supply. As a result, the CO_2 content of stack gases increases and CO content decreases. Free oxygen may pass through the coke bed, resulting in oxidation of iron and thus producing brown fumes discharging from the cupola stack. On the other hand, if the coke bed height is higher due to in sufficient air supply, the CO content of gases increases, which results in decrease of the metal temperature as well as the melting rate.

The coke bed height, the coke rate, air supply, the melting rate and the metal temperature, all are interrelated. These variables are very well related as shown by a typical 'Kite' or Net diagram[1] of Fig. 2.15. An examination of this diagram shows that in order to know the values of the two variables, one has to fix the other two. Thus, increasing the air volume increases the melting rate and raises the metal temperature for a constant iron-coke ratio. Faster melting is obtained because more coke is burnt producing more heat which in turn melts more metal. The temperature of the metal is raised because the proportion of the total heat lost through cupola walls is less with fast melting and hence, iron must be hotter. A decrease in the iron-coke ratio means an increase in the relative amount of coke. Therefore, the melting rate decreases with constant air supply. The metal temperature increases with a decrease in the iron-coke ratio because more heat is developed per unit of the metal. Different types of such diagrams are required to be developed for different sizes of the cupola.

The coke rate or coke consumption is an important parameter determining the economics of the cupola operation. A number of the following factors determine this parameter :

(*i*) The design of cupola
(*ii*) The quality of the coke (i.e. ash content of the coke)
(*iii*) The amount of the steel scrap in the charge
(*iv*) The size of the raw materials

(*v*) The quality of pig iron used (i.e. its phosphorus content)

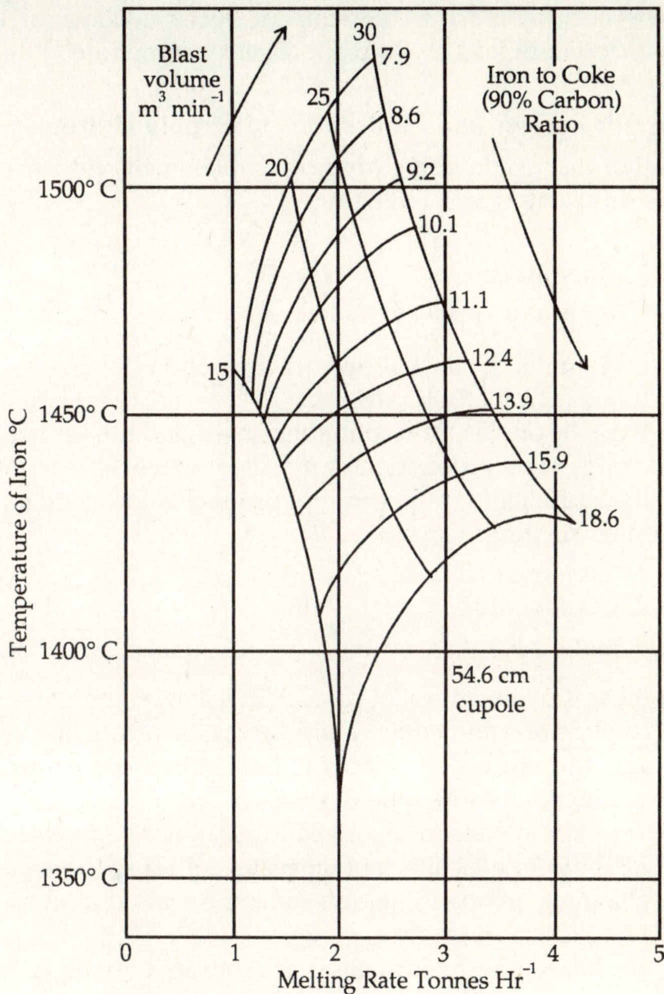

Fig. 2.15: A Net Diagram Showing Relationship between Air Blast Rates, Iron to Coke Ratios, Metal Temperatures and Melting Rates[1] (Courtesy of Portcullis Press, Redhill).

A high-phosphorus pig iron will require lower coke consumption due to formation of low melting eutectic constituent. Similarly, small pieces of pig iron will melt easily but small pieces of scrap oxidize fast and will require a higher coke rate. A higher percentage of scrap and a higher ash content of coke will lead to more coke consumption. Besides the design of a conventional cupola, a number of modifications in the cupola design such as use of preheated blast, O_2 enrichment, water cooling of cupola etc. will certainly lead to different coke consumptions.

2.6.6 Advantages and Limitations of Cupola Melting

Like other cast iron melting furnaces, cupola melting furnace has also its advantages and limitations.

2.6.6.1 Advantages

The advantages of cupola are:

(*i*) It is simple in construction and operation.
(*ii*) It has high melting rates.
(*iii*) It can be operated on continuous basis and thus suitable for a large scale production of metal over an extended period.
(*iv*) Its equipment cost per unit of product is lower than many other melting furnaces.

2.6.6.2 Disadvantages

Against above advantages, cupola has the following limitations :

(*i*) It has limited control of composition and temperature. Both composition and temperature vary widely from heat to heat and therefore, the cupola is best suited for continuous production of one type of iron.
(*ii*) The carbon content of cupola iron can not be reduced to < 2.8% due to the contact of the metal with coke in the hearth.
(*iii*) The metal temperature also can not be raised to more than 1450° C.
(*iv*) Oxidation and melting loses are considerably high.

Inspite of these disadvantages, cupola still remains the major primary melting furnace, particularly for melting of gray and alloy cast irons. The cupola can be also used for duplex melting along with other furnaces like rotary furnaces, direct arc and coreless induction furnaces for melting of special cast irons.

3

Modern Developments in Cupola Melting Practice

3.1 INTRODUCTION

Although the conventional acid lined cold blast cupola has been the traditional melting unit in the foundry industry ever since its inception, over the last 7-8 decades, a number of developments have taken place in cupola melting of cast irons which have been adopted with varying degree of success. Many refinements and modifications in the form of mechanization and the addition of numerous accessories have been introduced. The aim of such developments have been to improve the performance and efficiency of cupola melting so as to obtain greater economy by increased production and reduced energy consumption. Another major purpose of the many of above modifications has been to extend the range of usefulness of the cupola for cast iron melting.

In addition to the use of greater mechanization and automation in cupola charging, adoption of cupola fore hearth and continuous slagging and tapping operations, various other major developments which have taken place can be enumerated as :

1. Use of preheated blast or Hot blast operation
2. Use of cupola water cooling or Lining less cupola operation
3. Basic slag cupola operation or Basic slag cupola melting
4. Balanced blast or Divided blast cupola operation
5. Use of oxygen in cupola
6. Use of supplementary fluxes in cupola melting
7. Use of supplementary fuels in cupola
8. Use of plasma arc in cupola melting
9. Cokeless cupola or Gas fired cupola melting
10. Use of increased cupola well depth

11. Post-melting cupola metal treatments
12. Use of computers in cupola operation

The details of each of above developments may be discussed as follows.

3.2 HOT BLAST CUPOLA OPERATION

One of the early and most prominent developments which took place in the early of 1950's and which is most extensively applied throughout the world has been the introduction of cupola air blast preheating. The simple reason to heat the cupola air supply is to save coke consumption since the combustion flame temperature increases which inturn increases the melting rate and the tapping temperature and thereby there is increase in the solubility of carbon in the iron. Associated with this is the lower sulphure content of the metal due to use of less coke and decreased silicon loss due to higher tapping temperature which in turn makes practical the use of larger quantities of steel scrap in the charge. The coke which is soft or high in ash content can be also used because of support from recovered top gases.

Approximately 55% of the heat generated in cupola melting is lost in the form of sensible heat and latent heat of the effluent gases escaping the cupola. This heat can be advantageously used in preheating the blast through recuperators usually upto 500° C. Fig. 3.1 summaries the results of the experiments conducted at a cupola plant of a premier cast iron research organization B.C.I.R.A.[2] illustrating the effect of preheated blast on the metal temperature and its composition when melting a given charge mixture. It is obvious from this figure that at a given coke charge, heating the air blast to 520° C increased the metal temperature by 100°C and increased the carbon content of the metal tapped by 0.4%. The silicon content of the metal was also increased and the sulphur pick-up was reduced. With a cold blast operation, a coke charge of 16% was required to obtain a metal temperature of 1520° C. When the blast was preheated to 520°C the same metal temperature could be obtained at a coke charge of 10.7%. It is obvious that the effect of hot blast in increasing the carbon pick-up will enable pig iron of the charge to be replaced by steel scrap. In addition, the reduced sulphur content of the metal will permit a higher proportion of cast iron scrap to be incorporated in the cupola charges. Such replacements in the charge constituents may substantially beneficially affect the cost of materials used in the cupola.

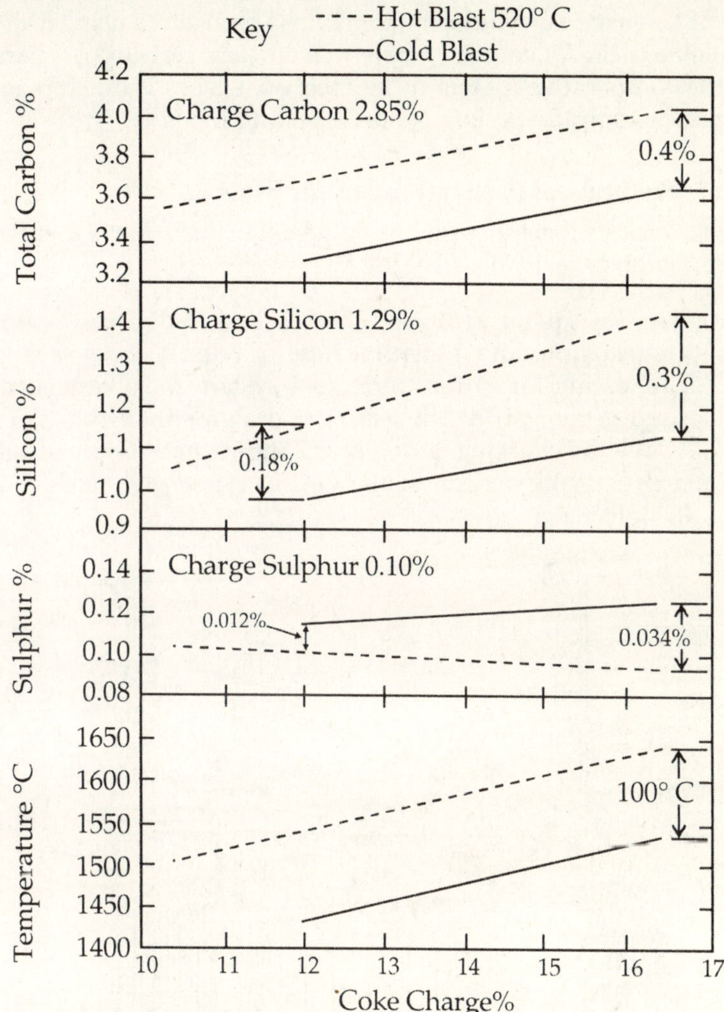

Fig. 3.1: Effect of preheated blast on cupola metal composition and temperature

It is now well established that the economic benefits diminish when the blast temperature is raised much in excess of 500° C since recuperators for operation at higher temperatures become unduly expensive. Further, as the capital cost of installing preheated facilities will be high, the use of hot blast operation is only justified for cupolas of greater capacities, particularly operated on continuous basis. However, small foundries may make use of less expensive independently fired preheaters using locally available fuels. Of course, the thermal efficiency of cupolas based on the recuperative system using their own gases is much higher than those employing independent heating methods.

3.2.1 Methods of Preheating the Air Blast

The air blast is generally preheated to 400 to 500° C and there are three methods normally used for the same.

(*i*) **The Recuperative Type:** This method makes use of both the sensible and potential heat of cupola top gases for preheating air in recuperators-a system most extensively used in the world. The gases are drawn either from top or below the charging door. Fig. 3.2 shows an example of such a preheating system of the Griffin type[3], which is most widely used.

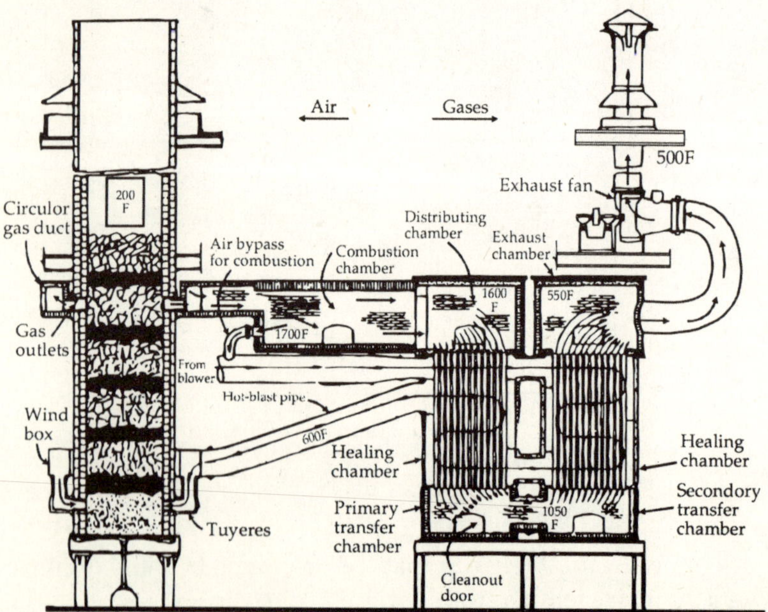

Fig. 3.2: Sectional view of hot-blast cupola of the Griffine type[3]

(*ii*) **The Modified Recuperative Type:** In this system only the sensible heat of the cupola gases is utilized. The gases are with drawn just above the melting zone.

(*iii*) **The Independently Fired Preheaters**: In such system, the preheaters are fired using locally available fuel like oil, gas or coal. The fuel is burnt in a combustion chamber and products pass over a tubular type heat exchanger. The main advantages of such externally fired units is that their operation is independent of cupola effluent gas analyzes and thus does not require control of cupola charges. At the same time, the temperature of the preheated gas can be better controlled.

The choice between above systems of preheating the blast depends upon the relative capital costs of the systems used and on the prices and availability of the coke and of the alternate fuels. Separately fired preheaters use fuels other than the coke used for cupola operation, coke of poor quality or other locally available in expensive fuels.

3.2.2 Advantages of Hot Blast Operation

Various advantages which can be obtained by use of preheated blast are:

(*i*) Reduced coke consumption (by 30 to 40%) and increased melting rate
(*ii*) For the same coke rate, a higher pouring or tapping temperature
(*iii*) Increased carbon pick-up and therefore increased use of steel scrap
(*iv*) Reduced sulphur pick-up and increased silicon-pick due to increased melt temperature
(*v*) Reduced melting losses
(*vi*) Permits use of low grade coke, i.e. soft or high ash coke
(*vii*) Better cupola operation due to less tendency to bridging and tuyere plugging

3.2.3 Limitations of Hot Blast Operation

Against the above advantages, the following are disadvantages :

(*i*) Increased capital and maintenance costs and therefore economical for large capacity cupolas running on continuous basis
(*ii*) High rate of lining erosion
(*iii*) Greater control of equipment required

3.3 USE OF WATER COOLING OR LININGLESS CUPOLA OPERATION

Shortly after introduction of hot-blast, a need for reducing refractory consumption and extending the melting campaigns was felt and this led to development of the use of water cooling of cupola lining. Besides minimizing the consumption of refractories in various operating zones, water cooling of the cupola is also adopted for the following reasons:

(*i*) To extend the duration of a melting heat
(*ii*) To reduce the labour and time required for repairing the lining
(*iii*) To reduce the consumption of expensive basic refractory materials
(*iv*) To enable the internal diameter of cupola to be increased by reducing the lining thickness or removing the lining completely in the melting zone so that a higher melting rate may be obtained.
(*v*) To stabilize the inside diameter of cupola to give a constant coke burning area and hence, a much more uniform and predictable operation.

3.3.1 Limitations of Water Cooling

Against the above advantages, a major disadvantage of water cooling is the reduction in the metal temperature or alternatively, an increase in the coke consumption to obtain a certain desired temperature. This effect becomes increasingly serious as the cupola diameter decreases. This is for the reason that the heat transmitted to the cooling water depends on the area of the cooling surface which is directly proportional to the cupola diameter. However, the heat developed by the combustion of the coke depends on the cross-sectional area of the melting zone and this is proportional to the square of the cupola diameter. The fraction of the total heat developed which is abstracted by the cooling water therefore diminishes as the cupola diameter increases. This is obvious from the Fig. 3.3 which shows relationship between the cupola diameter and the heat loss to the water cooled shell of a cupola for a 2 metre water cooled height[4]. For this reason, it is not generally advisable to water cool cupolas of less than 900 mm internal diameter especially if high tapping temperatures are required. Besides reduction in metal temperature, the capital cost of a water cooled cupola is of course, higher than that of a conventional cupola. However, if water is available, this higher cost may be compensated by savings in refractory material and labour cost incurred in repairing and maintenance.

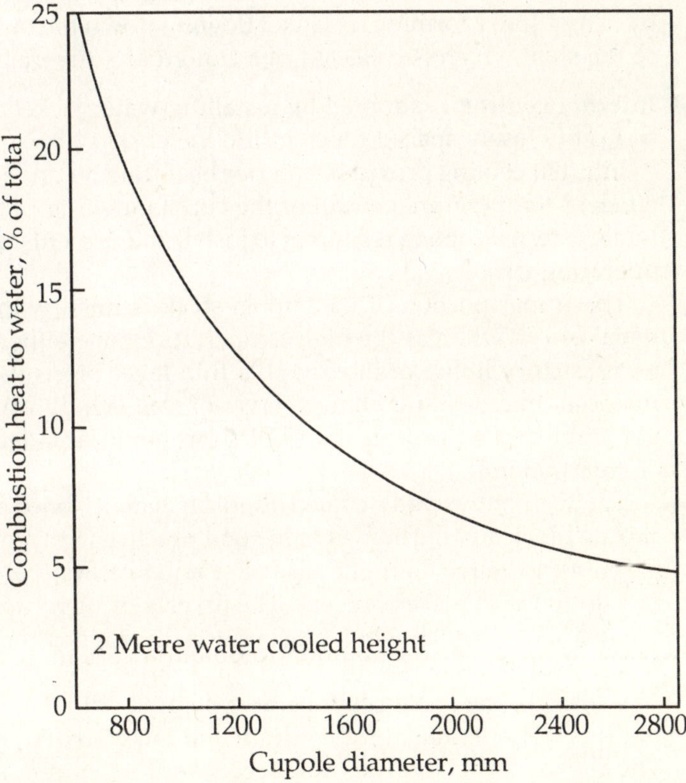

Fig. 3.3: Relation between heat loss to cooling water and cupola diameter

3.2.2 Methods of Water Cooling

In order to keep heat loss to water at a minimum, the height of the water cooled zone has been decreased in recent past years. The zone of maximum temperature in a cupola extends only a metre or so above the tuyere level and water cooling is therefore of real advantage for cooling a height of only a metre or two at the most.

The amount of water used for cooling varies greatly in practice depending on the height of the water cooled zone, temperature rise permitted in the water, the cost of water and the confidence of the operator. A practical figure to use water for the design of a 2 metre height is 35 litres per cm of cupola circumference.

Two methods of water cooling is adopted as described below:

(*i*) **External cooling** in which the cupola shell is water cooled by heavy spray forming a blanket flowing down the outside of the shell which is collected in a trough at a tuyere level.

(*ii*) **Internal cooling** is adopted by installing water jackets or a series of closely spaced tubes inside the cupola shell.

Internal cooling provides superior heat transfer and more efficient temperature control of the cupola melting process while external cooling is simpler to install and presents fewer operating problems.

The upper portion of the cupola stack is lined with the usual bricks whereas the high temperature zone either has no refractory lining or lined with a thin layer of insulating material. In case of no lining, a layer of slag is built up and get stabilized to protect the shell from being abraded by charge material.

The well of the water cooled cupola is usually lined with carbon block and the lining life in good practice with regular patching is better than one year. Rammed carbon patches are also used in place of blocks. The tuyeres of such cupolas are made of invariably of high conductivity copper and are water cooled.

Usually water cooled cupolas are operated with hot blast, but this is not essential for medium and large size cupolas. The above combination has now become quite common since water cooling facilitates the use of basic slag operation.

3.4 BASIC SLAG CUPOLA MELTING

A major limitation of conventional acid cupola melting is that it is not possible to reduce the sulphur content of the metal during melting. On the contrary, the metal always absorbs sulphur from the coke. To enable irons of low sulphur content to be produced, the slag must contain a high ratio of lime to silica and this requirement prohibits the use of acid refractories. The remedy is to use a basic cupola melting which has been developed due to above reasons. A basic cupola means that it has a basic lining in the melting zone (including oxidation and reduction zone) and well and the charge contains enough lime and magnesia to maintain a basic slag while melting. The slag basicity ratio (B) is variously expressed as:

$$B = \frac{CaO + MgO}{SiO_2 + Al_2O_3}$$

or

$$= \frac{CaO + MgO}{SiO_2}$$

or

$$\text{Simply} = \frac{CaO}{SiO_2}$$

The value of B for basic melting practice should be > 1.3 in comparison to acid melting practice in which it varies between 0.3 to 0.5. In basic cupola melting, besides the basic slag, the furnace lining is that of magnesite and/or dolomite bricks backed by firebrick lining and this basic lining extends 5 to 10 feet above the tuyere level whereas rest lining is acid.

One of the advantagesof operating a basic cupola is that the steel scrap may be the only raw material used as the metallic charge. The use of such a large amount of steel scrap is possible because the basic slag fluxes the ash of the coke and makes a relatively large amount of carbon available for combination with the iron. Such carbon pick-up may be as high as 2 to 2.5%. Another associated advantage of this melting may be that the use of such a large amount of steel scrap (which will be low in phosphorus) will produce low phosphorus iron. However, the silicon loss will be quite high as high as 35 to 40% against 10% loss in acid melting. Such a high loss not only makes FeSi addition necessary but it will also produce more SiO_2 which reduces the basicity of slag. The remedy is to use the preheated blast which will reduce the silicon loss during melting and thus less SiO_2 is formed to reduce the slag basicity.

In order to achieve the required degree of basicity of slag, a larger percentage of flux is used in basic cupola melting than the acid melting. Thus, the acid melting fluxing cost is much lower than basic melting fluxing cost. Besides the main flux material i.e. the lime stone, a secondary flux such as fluor spar (CaF_2) is also necessary to increase the fluidity of the slag so that the large quantity of the slag produced does not become too viscous to remove it from the cupola.

When an excess of basic oxides like CaO, MgO etc. is available in the charge, the desulphurization reaction in basic cupola melting occurs under the reducing condition as:

$$C + CaO + \underline{S} \rightarrow CaS + Fe + CO$$

$$C + MgO + \underline{S} \rightarrow MgS + Fe + CO$$

The basic oxide MgO is less effective than CaO in desulphurization of the metal and hence, a high calcium limestone is preferred than a dolomatic stone as the flux material. The CaS and/or MgS formed in the above reaction leave the cupola in the form of slag.

The basic cupola operation consumes at least 50% more lining than does the acid cupola. Not that the basic refractories are costlier than the acid ones, even their patching materials are also costlier. Moreover, the magnesite bricks as the lining material have shorter life than the acid firebricks. As such, the use of basic linings in cupola creates a number of difficulties due to high rate of wear of the material, its expense and the general difficulty of carrying out lining repairs. The solutions to these problems have been generally implemented in the forms of water cooling of the high temperature zone which may be completely unlined or provided internally with a thin refractory lining which soon stabilizes itself against the slag attack owing to the action of the cooling water. The well of such cupola is sometimes provided with a neutral lining for slags of only moderate basicity but for highly basic slags, a carbon lining is generally used.

Water cooling in basic slag operation is justified in view of the metallurgical and economic benefits obtained but the coke consumption is generally higher than acid practice. The use of preheated blast along with water cooling therefore can take care of the both the silicon loss and high coke consumption of the basic slag operation and this combination is practiced in new cupola installations.

It is well established that the effect of increasing the slag basicity is to reduce sulphur content and increase the carbon content of the metal while silicon loss is increased. Figs. 3.4 and 3.5 show the effect of slag basicity on metal composition in terms of S, C and Si contents and the metal temperature at a constant coke charge, blast rate and blast temperature for a lining less melting zone (high temperature zone) and a carbon lined well of a cupola[4]. It may be seen that at higher sulphur levels i.e. when operating with an acid slag, considerable latitude exists to enable the carbon content to be varied (Fig. 3.4) over quite a wide range by appropriate selection of the operating conditions which influence the metal temperature. The extent to which it is possible to control the carbon content in this way diminishes as the basicity of the slag increases and the sulphur content decreases. At very low sulphur levels such as those desirable for production of S.G. irons, e.g. 0.01%, it is difficult to limit the carbon level to less than the eutectic content. Low carbon irons with low sulphur content can not therefore be produced from the basic cupola. On the other hand, high carbon irons of low sulphur content can be produced from high steel charges. The required silicon content is obtained by adding ferrosilicon to the charge.

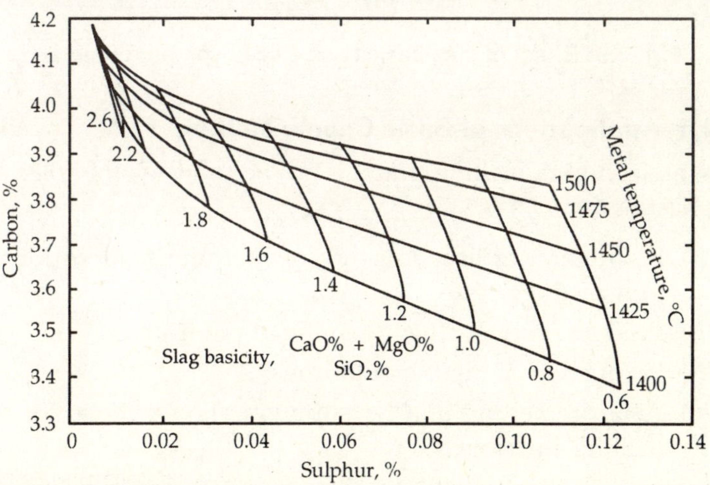

Fig. 3.4: Relationship between carbon and sulphur contents of metal, slag basicity and metal temperature.

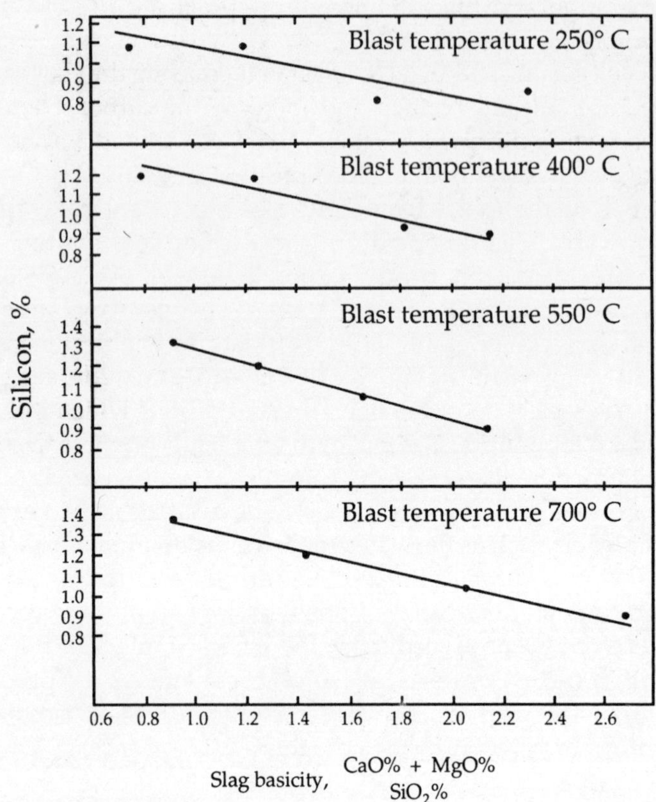

Fig. 3.5: Effect of slag basicity on silicon content of metal[5]

3.4.1 Applications of Basic Cupola Melting

The basic cupola melting practice can be used for the following applications:

(*i*) Production of base irons of low sulphur content for S.G. iron castings

(*ii*) Production of synthetic or refined pig irons

(*iii*) Production of ingot mould irons

(*iv*) As a premelting unit for supplying liquid metal for steel melting furnaces.

In all above cases, charges containing high proportions of steel scrap can be employed.

3.4.2 Advantages of Basic Cupola Melting

Such cupolas have the ability to use low cost charging materials consisting of as high as 100% steel charges to produce gray irons or other base irons that require low sulphur and/or low phosphorus with varying total carbon content.

3.4.3 Disadvantages of Basic Cupola Melting

Against the above advantages, the disadvantages are :

(*i*) Silicon losses are greater than in an acid cupola melting
(*ii*) Refractory costs are 2 to 3 times that of an acid cupola
(*iii*) Cost of fluxing material is higher than that of acid cupola
(*iv*) More coke consumption and hence, slower melting rate than acid cupola when operated with cold blast
(*v*) Metal analysis is more difficult to control than acid cupola.

The use of water cooling along with hot blast operation can take care of many of the above limitations of basic slag cupola melting.

3.5 USE OF BALANCED BLAST OR DIVIDED BLAST OPERATION

A number of claims have been made in the past that the performance and operation of a cupola can be significantly improved by the introduction of the blast air through two or more rows of tuyeres. Thus, the Balanced Blast Cupola was developed in 1930 in U.K. which was based on the principle of balancing the rate of air supply between the lower and upper rows of tuyeres and substantial coke savings were claimed. However, consistently good results could not be obtained due to the inability to measure and control the air flow individually to each row of tuyeres although some cupolas of this type are still in operation.

Later on, researches have established that the optimum number of rows of tuyeres are two and it is believed that the air admitted to the upper row of tuyeres burns the carbon mono-oxide formed in gases ascending the cupola shaft to carbon dioxide, thus releasing virtually all of the potential heat of the coke charged.

BCIRA conducted a series of tests[6] to establish the optimum conditions for a cupola operating with two row of tuyeres. The experiments were carried out with a cupola of 760 mm internal diameter with two rows of tuyeres (Fig. 3.6) to which air was supplied from a separate wind belt and the blast to each row were measured, recorded and controlled. Effect of varying the distribution of blast between the lower and upper row of tuyeres and spacings in between these rows were studied for different conditions of the blast rate and coke charges. It was established by these experiments that the 50% of the total blast be admitted through each row of tuyeres and there was an optimum spacing (900 mm) between the two rows of these tuyeres to give the best results. Any deviations from these conditions led to decrease in metal temperature.

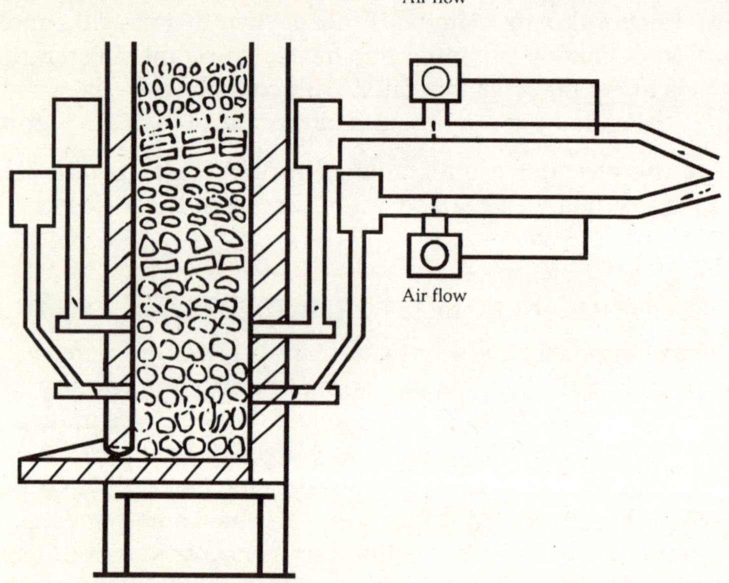

Fig. 3.6: Diagramatic representation of a divided blast cupola

Fig. 3.7 clearly shows that compared with operation of a cupola with one row of tuyeres, the use of two rows of tuyeres at an optimum spacing of 900 mm with the blast equally divided resulted in an increase of 45 to 50° C in the tapping temperature with the same coke rate. It is obvious from this figure that at a coke charge of 15%, a tapping temperature of 1500° C would be obtained using one row of tuyeres or 1545° C using two rows of tuyeres.

In most foundries, a given tapping temperature is normally required. The above figure shows the extent to which coke charge could be reduced for a given metal temperature. For example, for a metal temperature of 1500° C, a coke charge of 15% in one row cupola operation will be reduced to 10.8% when using two rows of tuyeres. The corresponding melting rate increase will be 19% and the coke consumption will be reduced by 28%. Depending on the level of the metal temperature required, the divided blast operation enables coke charge consumption to be reduced by 20 to 32% and the melting rate will be increased by 11 to 23%.

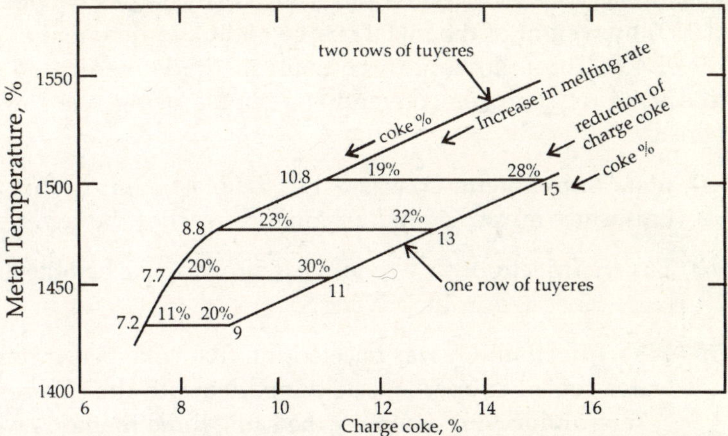

Fig. 3.7: Variation of metal temperature with percentage of coke charge for one row and two rows of tuyeres operation

With divided blast operation, there is an extension of the operating height of the coke bed further up the furnace shaft and the depth of the superheating zone in the furnace is also increased. However, there is not much change in the metal composition. The increase in metal temperature due to divided blast operation will also lead to increase in carbon pick-up and thereby enabling foundries to increase the proportion of steel scrap in the charge.

There are a large number of cupolas operating with divided blast in U.K. The above successful operation has also led to installation of divided blast cupolas throughout the would including USA, Canada, France and Japan.

3.6 USE OF OXYGEN IN CUPOLAS

Interest in the use of oxygen in cupola in recent past years has increased due to increase in metal temperature, production rate and carbon pick-up. The increase in metal temperature is possible due to the fact that the use of O_2 increases the combustion temperature in the high temperature zone like the use of preheated blast and in this respect, use of one per cent O_2 has the same effect as obtained by preheating the blast by ~ 85° C.

BCIRA has studied in detail to determine the effects of using oxygen in the conventional cupola and in the divided blast cupola. Tests were made[6] with a cupola of 760 mm internal diameter at a constant blast rate of 43 Nm^3/min using coke charges between 7 and 15% by weight of the metal charge and O_2 enrichment at the level of 4%. The following three main methods were used for introducing oxygen in a conventional cupola using one row of tuyeres:

(*i*) **Blast Enrichment:** O_2 was fed to the blast main so that the uniformly mixed O_2 and air mixture reaches the tuyeres .

(*ii*) **Tuyere Injection:** O_2 was injected into the coke bed through lances inserted in the tuyeres.

(*iii*) **Well Injection:** O_2 was injected into the coke bed through water cooled copper lances located beneath the tuyeres.

In a divided blast cupola, the same three methods were used and enrichment to both rows of tuyeres were investigated and in case of tuyere injection, lances were inserted through the bottom row of tuyeres only.

Fig. 3.8 shows the effects of the above three methods on relation between the metal temperature and the coke charge for both conventional and divided blast operations. As obvious from the curve in above figure, the increase in metal tapping temperature in divided blast operation was obtained as compared with conventional operation without oxygen. The increases in metal temperature using the three methods of oxygen were as follows:

Conventional Operation:

Enrichment of the blast

+ 50° C

Tuyere injection

+ 40° C

Well injection – 230 mm below tuyeres

+ 50° C

– 610 mm below tuyeres

+ 85° C

– 910 mm below tuyeres

+ 85° C

Divided-blast Operation:

Without oxygen

+ 50° C

Enrichment-lower row of tuyeres

+ 85° C

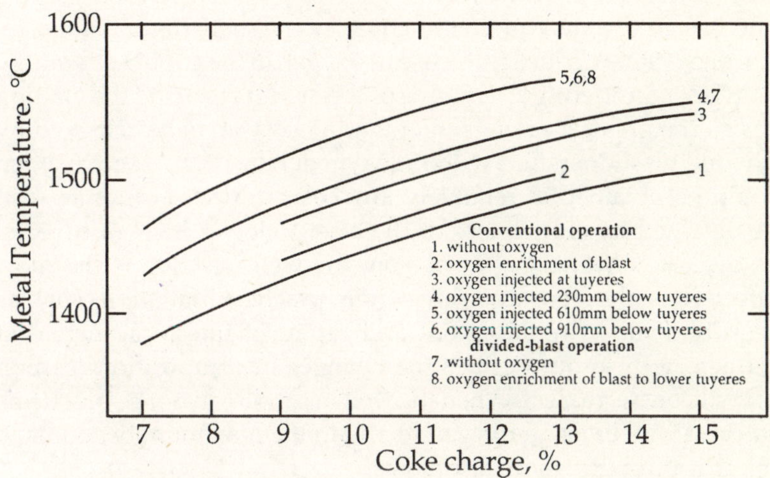

Fig. 3.8: Variation of metal temperature with percentage of coke charge for different methods of oxygen enrichment in conventional and devided blast operations.

It is obvious from the above data that in case of conventional operation, simple enrichment of the blast was the least efficient method of using oxygen in the cupola whereas the well injection was the most effective in increasing the metal temperature. Of course, the maximum effective distance of injection from tuyeres was 610 mm. In case of divided blast operation, maximum metal temperature at any given coke charge, was obtained when oxygen was used to enrich the blast supplied to lower row of tuyeres. This method of operation increased the tapping temperature by 85° C above those of conventional operation and 35° C above those obtained in divided blast operation without oxygen. The use of tuyere injection and well injection did not produce any better results than blast enrichment of last row of tuyeres.

It was also found that the melting rate increased when the coke charge decreased. Thus, in foundries, where is requirement of the metal at a given temperature, these methods of oxygen injection are quite coke saving and increasing the melting rate. It was possible for a 1500° C metal temperature, to reduce coke consumption from 15% to 8% for divided blast operation and increase the melting rate by 46% with oxygen enrichment of the blast. Thus, increased melting rates obtained by the use of oxygen, divided blast operation or both together can produce considerable economic benefit. However, in view of the high cost of oxygen, one has to decide whether such economic benefits obtained by use of oxygen will justify the use of oxygen in the cupola operation.

When considering alternative processes for reducing the melting costs, the greatest savings in operating costs may be achieved by divided blast operation without oxygen. However, where oxygen could be obtained at relatively low costs, further economies can be obtained by enrichment of the blast to lower level of tuyeres. In case of conventional operation, the well injection is the most effective method but there are certain practical limitations such as requirements of replacement and repair of injectors, increased refractory burn out besides the changes in composition (carbon and silicon decreases). When the well injection can not be practiced, the best way of using oxygen to obtain the maximum benefit is to inject it through lances at tuyeres.

3.7 USE OF SUPPLEMENTARY FLUXES

An addition of limestone is normally made in cupola charges in order to flux the ash of the coke, eroded refractory and certain oxidation products formed during melting. In a cold blast acid lined cupola operation, this addition is of the order of 3% of the metal charged or may be higher in some practices. The above flux addition may be supplemented in one of a number of different proprietary fluxing briquettes such as those based on either fluorspar (CaF_2) or soda ash (Na_2CO_3) which are marketed with the claims that they improve the slag fluidity permitting easier tapping of the slag with other benefits such as improved carbon pick-up and reduced sulphur content of the tapped metal.

BCIRA conducted[6] a series of tests to study the effects of such additions to supplement or replace an existing limestone addition using the divided blast cupola operation at a constant coke rate of 11% and using 3% limestone. Fig. 3.9 shows the effects of addition of such supplementary fluxes on carbon and sulphur contents of the metal tapped. It was found that the addition of fluorspar increased the carbon pick-up upto 1% fluorspar addition and after that no increase in carbon pick-up was noticed. The increase in limestone addition did not produce any significant change whereas the soda ash decreased gradually the carbon content of the metal. It was also found that the sulphur content reduced by increasing the addition of the flux but the use of soda ash or fluorspar did not cause any greater reduction than that which could be achieved by the use of an equivalent quantity of limestone.

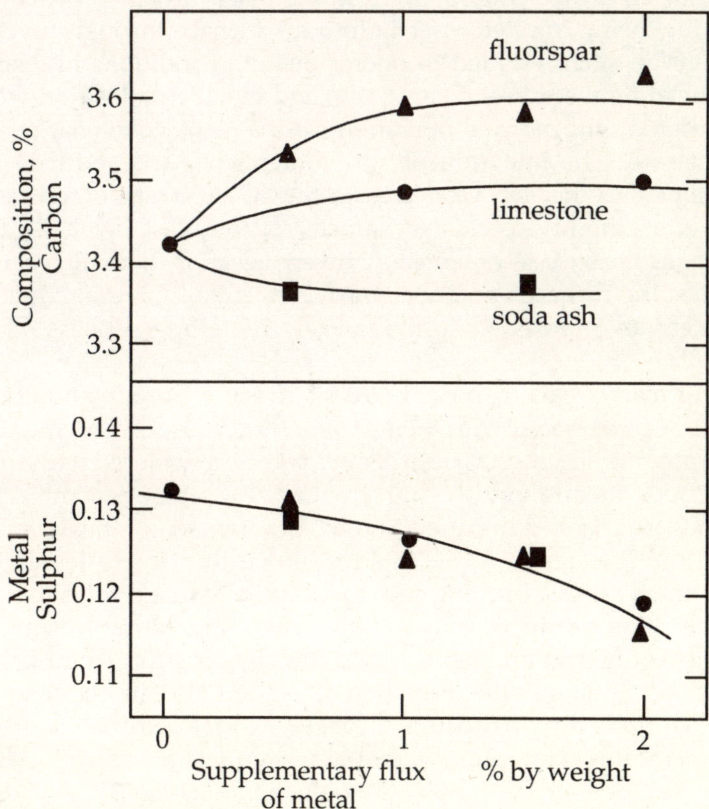

Fig. 3.9: Effects of additions of supplementary fluxes on metal composition

Hence, the above results show that significant increase in carbon pick-up could be obtained when upto 1% fluorspar is used to supplement the existing lime stone addition and thus more steel scrap can be used in the cupola charge. But when higher flux addition causes more refractory consumption, it will be better to use fluorspar to replace part of the limestone in the charge rather than to supplement it.

3.8 USE OF SUPPLEMENTARY FUELS

In the recent past years, considerable interest has been aroused in the possibility of partially replacing the coke in cupolas with lower cost fuels. Early tests with such supplementary fuels were conducted on the line followed in the blast furnace practice i.e., the fuel being injected directly into the furnace through tuyeres. However, such tests led to poorer melting conditions in respect of metal temperature, melting rate and metal composition when compared with normal operation for the same coke charge and blast rate. The injection of supplementary fuels reduced the combustion efficiency i.e. decreased the CO_2/CO ratio of top gases. The more highly reducing character of the blast furnace gases explains the success obtained by tuyere injection of auxiliary fuels in the blast furnace operation which is essentially an ore reduction process as opposed to almost purely remelting process of the cupola.

For many years, cupolas in Russia, Eastern Europe and U.S.A. have been operated with the use of natural gas as supplementary fuel and the success has been claimed. They considered it essential that such fuels should be burnt with air in separate combustion chambers attached to cupola and the products of combustion pass into the furnace at 1 to 2 metres above the tuyere level. The argument against burning such fuels at the tuyere level is that the combustion products, CO_2 and H_2O react unfavourably with the hot coke in the combustion zone thereby reducing combustion efficiency owing to the formation of CO and H_2. The reduction of the combustion products proceeds more rapidly at high temperatures. However, when these products are introduced at a higher level in the cupola, the reduction does not take place to such an extent as it does at the tuyere level since the temperature at such level is lower. Therefore, the combustion efficiency is improved.

BCIRA also conducted a series of tests using oil and coke oven gases as supplementary fuels and a proportion of coke charge was replaced by the thermal equivalent of the gas or oil. However, the conclusion was that no reduction in the overall fuel consumption could be achieved by the use of such fuels and the high tapping temperature could not be achieved. Nevertheless, some foundries in U.K. still use coke oven gas as supplementary fuel and considerable reduction in coke consumption have been reported for cases where high tapping temperatures are not required.

3.9 USE OF PLASMA ARC IN CUPOLA MELTING

In the recent past, attempt has been made[7] to use the plasma torch in cupola melting with the aim to obtain saving in coke consumption. Experiments were conducted in a pilot plant cupola in 1982 at Pittsbergh, USA and very encouraging results were obtained. Figure 3.10 shows schematic of such a plasma-fired cupola. In a water cooled plasma torch arc was produced

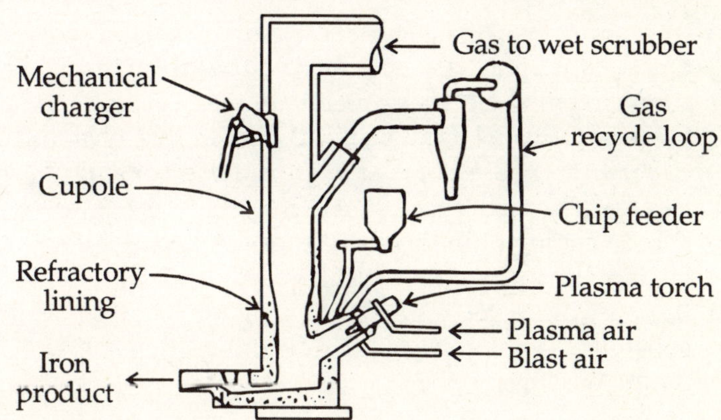

Fig. 3.10: Schematic of a plasma-fired pilot cupola (Reprinted with permission of ASM International)

by passing a high intensity direct current between two copper sleeves through the space in which air was introduced and ionized to produce very high temperatures in the melting zone of the furnace. The arc is rotated by a magnetic field. The temperatures produced were almost double or more than the maximum temperature produced by burning any fuel. The melting rate was found to be increased by 50% leading to considerable saving in coke consumption. Since the air blast was passed at low velocity, very fine charge components like turnings and borings could be used in the charge, as high as 70% of the charge. The cupola also produced less oxidizing gas with low velocity effluent coming out of the cupola. The experiments showed that it was possible to use very high metal to coke ratio as high as 70 : 1 against the conventional cupola operation using 5 to 15 : 1. Such a cupola development has also led to commercial plants installed and in operation in earlie's of 1990. However, one has to work out the economics of such a operation against the savings in coke consumption obtained. It is claimed that it is possible to use low grade coke and other fuels such as coke breeze or anthracite coal in place of the coke required for a normal cupola operation.

3.9.1 Advantages of Plasma Fired Cupolas

The following advantages have been claimed by use of such cupolas:

(*i*) Coke consumption can be considerably reduced by supplementing electric power from the plasma torch.

(*ii*) Lower-quality coke can be used. Besides this, blast furnace coke, fine waste coke and anthracite coal have been successfully used.

(*iii*) Direct melting of borings and turnings is possible.

(*iv*) High metal to coke ratio can be used.

(*v*) It is possible to get iron reduced from iron oxide and silicon generated by injecting iron oxide and sand, respectively at the tuyere level.

3.10 COKELESS CUPOLAS OR GAS FIRED CUPOLAS

A final attempt to completely eliminate the use of coke in cupola melting was made in the 1970s in U.K. and a so-called "cokeless cupola" was developed[8] fired with gas or oil. Such cupolas are also called 'Gas fired' cupolas and they are in operation in several countries of the world.

Figure 3.11 shows a schematic sketch of such a cupola which is a refractory-lined shaft furnace with a water cooled steel pipe grate supporting a bed of refractory lumps or spheres and is placed above the burners. This bed of refractory spheres is used to support the metal to be melted. The heat for melting and superheating is generated by either gas or oil burners placed equally spaced round the circumference of the cupola. As the metal melts, it gets superheated while passing through the refractory bed and collected in the well and is tapped as required. The tapping temperature obtained is about 1450° C. Some loss of carbon occurs during melting and so to obtain the required carbon content in the metal, a carburizing agent (petroleum coke or graphite) is injected into the well just below the burner level above the slag.

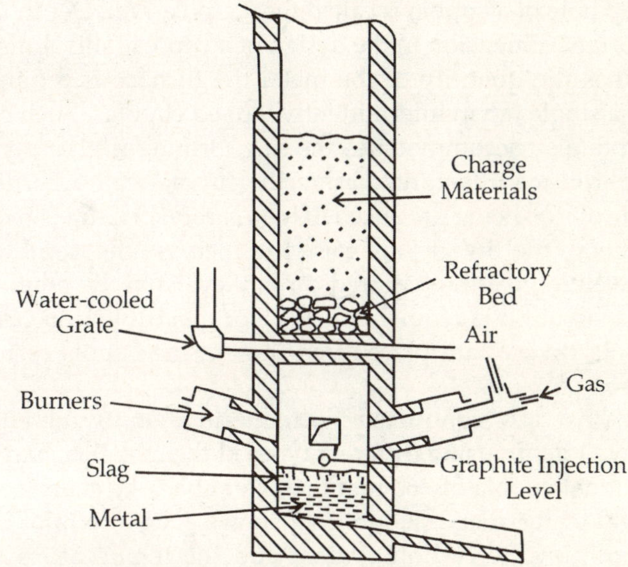

Fig. 3.11: Schematic sketch of a cokeless cupola

The advantages of using such cupolas are:

(*i*) Low dust content of the effluent gas, makes the exhaust gas virtually invisible and thus pollution is minimal and would meet environmental standards without expensive emission control equipment.

(*ii*) SO_2 content of the exhaust gas is also very lower than that of coke-fired cupolas.

(*iii*) The sulphur pick up by the metal is very low (as low as 0.01% S) making such melting unit of great interest for foundries producing S.G. iron.

As such, in the countries, where a coke is imported at a high price and the gas or oil is readily available, such a cokeless cupola is economically very attractive. Several small cupolas of 5 to 10 tons/hour capacity are in operation in several countries of the world. However, the high cost of the refractory sphere replacement and the restrictions on the percentage of steel scrap used are the major limitations of such cupolas.

3.11 USE OF INCREASED CUPOLA WELL DEPTH

The vertical distance between the centre of tuyeres to the centre of the tap hole of a cupola is called the 'Cupola Well Depth' and is an important dimension in the design of a cupola. This dimension determines the quantity of the metal the furnace is required to yield in a single tap in intermittently tapped cupolas. Such cupola well depth also accommodates the slag forming in that period.

Some iron manufactures design the cupola well according to the grade of iron being produced. If high carbon pick-up is required in the metal, the tuyeres are raised to increase the depth of the cupola well to give the required carbon level. On the other hand, if low-carbon iron is required such as for malleable iron castings, the cupola tuyeres are placed very low in the cupola to restrict the carbon pick-up.

BCIRA has also conducted[6] some tests to study the effect of cupola well depth using different types of the metallic charge in a conventional cupola of 760 mm diameter at a coke charge of 15% by weight of the metal. Figure 3.12 shows such effects of cupola well depth on the carbon content and the temperature of the tapped metal. As is obvious from this figure, with both kinds of charge, the tapped carbon content was raised by increasing the well depth, the increase being equivalent to 0.13 and 0.43 per cent for the high- and low-carbon charges, respectively, for each metre increase in the well depth. The well depth did not affect the Si, Mn, S and P contents of the metal. However, the metal temperature was reduced by approximately 31° C per metre increase in the well depth due to heat lost to refractories in the well.

Such ability to increase carbon pick-up by extending the well depth of a cupola offers foundries the opportunity to substitute steel scrap for pig-iron in the charge producing a given grade of iron. In many countries, the economic benefits of such substitution may considerably out weigh the cost of any additional charge coke needed to maintain a given tapping temperature.

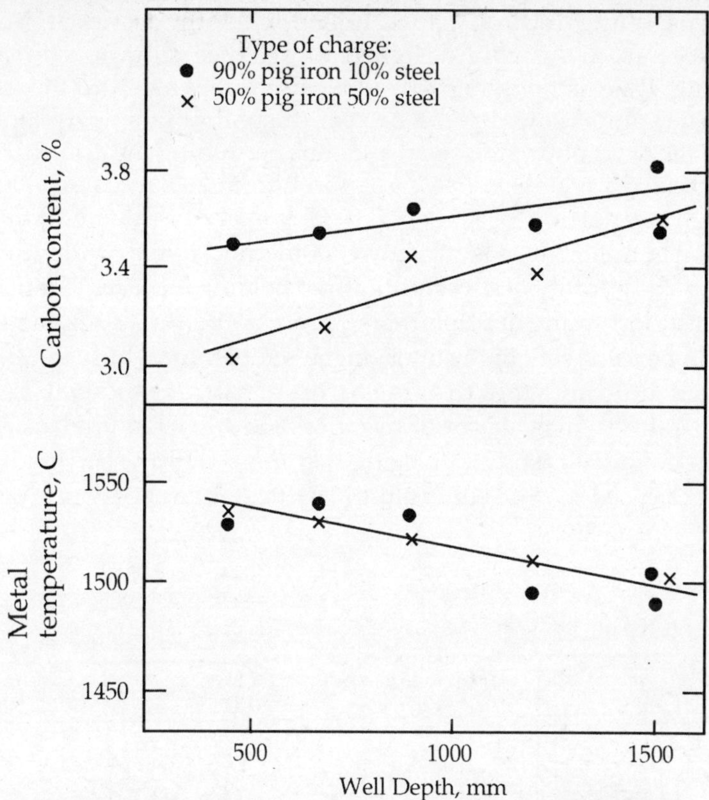

Fig. 3.12: Effects of cupola well depth on the carbon content and temperature of the tapped metal

3.12 POST-MELTING CUPOLA METAL TREATMENTS

Conventional cold blast and acid cupola melting is unable to reduce the sulphur content of the metal and the remedy for the same was sought in form of the basic cupola melting. However, the basic cupola melting is not only expensive to operate and maintain but it also leads to high silicon losses and produces an enatially high carbon content in the iron. Therefore, for large scale operation, basic melting is now superseated by acid melting followed by one of a number of post cupola metal treatment processes developed [9] for desulphurization of the acid cupola metal. In all these processes (Fig. 3.13), the iron is mixed intimately with a desulphurizing agent such as calcium carbide, soda ash or quick lime. These processes, namely Shaking Ladle Method, Porous Plug Method, Lance Injection Method and Stirring Devices are invariably designed to produce agitation during mixing. It is also possible to add a carburizing agent to the iron such graphite, coke breeze or coal dust simultaneously along with the desulphurizing agent and thus permitting the acid cupola to produce a relatively low carbon iron from a charge containing a high proportion of steel scrap. However, as the solution of carbon in molten iron is strongly endothermic, it may be desirable to provide additional superheating and holding furnaces to replace the heat lost in the desulphurizing process and thus avoiding the need of excessively high cupola metal temperature. In such cases, such a holding unit provides iron of correct analysis and temperature which may be drawn up as and when required instead of the foundry casting rate being tied more rigidly. The holding furnaces used may be either electric induction furnaces or oil fired rotary furnaces.

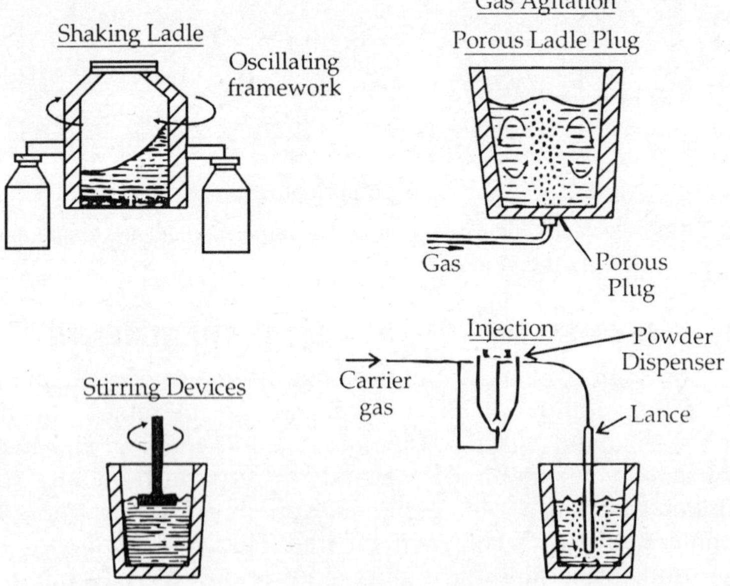

Fig. 3.13: Dust melting cupola metal treatment processes

All the above four methods of cupola metal treatment are also used for production of iron suitable for manufacture of S.G. cast irons.

The Shaking Ladle Method makes use of a rotary-reciprocating motion applied to the molten iron in the ladle so as to induce it to swirl with a parabolic meniscus. The ladle does not revolve about its own axis and such device produces a very efficient mixing during desulphurization. This equipment is suitable for treating large melts of several tons at a time for which the temperature loss is about one-quarter of that for small charges.

The Porus-Plug Method uses compressed air or nitrogen which is passed through a perforated refractory disc of the bottom of the treating vessel for bubling and mixing. Less temperature loss has been claimed for this method. In the Lance Injection Method, powdered materials such as calcium carbide, graphite, Fe-Si and other ferrous alloys, as may be needed, are blown through a graphite lance extending to near the bottom of the ladle by nitrogen gas under pressure. In the Stirring Devices, the agitation for mixing is produced by the rotation of impeller or propeller mixers specially designed for the same. All the above three methods are relatively simple, practical and inexpensive means for removal of sulphur from acid cupola metal.

3.13 USE OF COMPUTERS IN CUPOLA OPERATION

The ultimate refinement in a cupola operation is due to the use of the computers to record, monitor and control many of the important variables of cupola operation and such computer applications are continually being expanded.

Some of the most significant computer applications[10] are:

(*i*) Least cost cupola charge calculations by quickly calculating the charge cost of various combinations of suitable raw materials.

(*ii*) Metal weight compensation. In the dropping of the metal components from crane magnets into the weigh hoppers, any over shooting or under shooting can be balanced out by the computer on subsequent charges to be used.

(*iii*) Automatic weighing of coke, flux and ferrous alloys is done by computers.

(*iv*) Continuous analysis and recording of cupola top gas composition. In addition, alert signals are activated when explosive levels of hydrogen are approached from water leaks.

(*v*) Display of chemical analyses with statistical process control limits and alert signals when any element is approaching limits.

(*vi*) Indicating, recording or controlling of any data important to maintenance or control.

3.14 SELECTION OF A MELTING UNIT OR SYSTEM FOR CAST IRON MELTING

It is obvious from the previous chapter and the present chapter that there are a number of melting furnaces or combinations of such furnaces which can be selected for producing molten cast iron to meet the requirements of a particular foundry. However, there are a number of technical and economic factors which must be taken into account before a decision of the choice for a particular melting unit or system is made. The factors which must be considered are:

1. Volume and continuity of metal needed
2. Type (composition) of the metal or alloy to be melted
3. Melting and pouring temperature of the metal to be cast
4. Degree of metallurgical control (chemical and temperature control) required
5. Availability and relative casts of the metallic raw materials to be used
6. Availability and relative costs of the energy source required
7. Availability and the cost of the type of the labour required
8. Operating cost of the melting operation
9. Initial capital cost of the melting equipment required
10. Cleanliness and the noise level in operation

Of these factors, some are the constituents of the operating cost such as materials cost, cost of fuel or energy, cost of labour etc. but they are very much affected by the local factors and conditions and therefore, must be given due consideration separately in selection process.

Normally, it is difficult to give due importance to all the above factors and the selection of a melting unit or system is normally made based on consideration of a few important factors only.

As obvious from the characteristics, advantages and limitations of various furnaces available, no single type or simple combination of the melting units will be the best choice for all conditions of the material and energy source availability, type of metal required, pattern of demand and economic factors. All melting furnaces are suitable for a particular type of application. One can only weigh the merits and demerits of each type of melting unit/system and decide on the best choice he can make under the given set of circumstances and constraints.

To conclude, in general, the cupola has been the main melting unit used in iron foundries for many years for melting of the gray cast irons which account for the largest tonnage of cast irons produced. It still retains this commanding position even in the face of strong competition from the electric melting furnaces. The economics, working and the range of the utility of cupola melting have been considerably improved in the recent past years by several developments taken place and it is predicted that the modern cupola plants will continue to be used for medium and large scale gray iron production for some time to come. For example, in mechanized foundries, for large scale production of 10 to 20 tons/hour on continuous basis, there is no other option than cupolas.

The use of electric melting furnaces is continuously increasing in iron foundries due to their cleaner melting, versatility with respect to raw materials and products made and the degree of metallurgical control possible. For small scale production and quality requirements, the direct arc furnace and the coreless induction furnaces will be preferred. Mains frequency induction furnaces are most commonly employed and are under installation in new foundry units.

However, the furnaces operating at high frequencies have important advantages where a high concentration of power is required or where frequent changes of analysis to close specifications are necessary. High frequency furnaces are particularly useful in the latter applications.

For production of special cast irons like S.G. irons and malleable irons, in many cases a duplexing arrangement such as cupola + direct arc furnace, cupola + rotary furnace, cupola + mains frequency induction furnace, cupola + post metal treatment units etc. will be preferably used. The channel type induction furnaces will find increasing application for superheating and holding of irons melted in other furnaces provided that no major adjustment in composition is required.

Gray Cast Irons and Foundry Practice

4.1 INTRODUCTION

Of all the ferrous castings produced in the world, gray iron castings represent the largest tonnage manufactured by the foundry industries. The reasons for their popularity and extensive use of such castings are that gray cast irons are the least cost ferrous casting materials available which also combine excellent foundry characteristics with engineering properties like good machinability, high resistance to wear, good antifriction properties, high vibration damping capacity and high compression strength. All above characteristics of such casting alloys have led to their huge applications in automotive, truck, bus and tractor industries which alone accounts for a phenominal consumption of gray iron castings. In fact, the production of gray iron castings is twice annually to that of other cast metals combined. Similar reasons may be cited for their other applications such as sanitary castings and manhole covers, gas or water pipes for underground purposes, electric motor frames, machine tool structures (bases and supports), heat exchangers and radiators, ingot moulds, pistons rings, rolling mill and other general machinery parts.

In this chapter, it is proposed to discuss first the general metallurgy of gray cast irons dealing with their solidification behaviour, effects of process variables and composition on the morphology of graphite flakes formed and the properties of gray cast irons followed by different aspects of foundry practice used for production of such castings.

4.2 Fe-C-Si PHASE DIAGRAM AND SOLIDIFICATION OF FE-C-Si ALLOYS

Since the commercial gray cast irons contain significant amounts of silicon, a ternary phase diagram of the Fe-C-Si system can be discussed for the solidification behaviour of gray cast irons. The presence of silicon in such alloys is the most important single composition factor promoting graphitization in gray cast irons. The binary Fe-Fe_3C diagram is not a stable or equilibrium diagram and is rather a metastable diagram. The ternary Fe-C-Si system in which the second phase in the solid alloys is graphite is the equilibrium diagram. Fig. 4.1 is the vertical section of the ternary Fe-C-Si alloy system at 2% silicon[11] which has the appearance of a binary phase diagram and is also representative of the most commercial gray irons used. Therefore, it can be used for the present discussion of the solidification and transformation behaviour of gray irons.

As obvious from Fig. 4.1, the presence of 2% silicon in gray iron changes in the extent and positions of the regions of the Fe-Fe_3C binary diagram in the following respects:

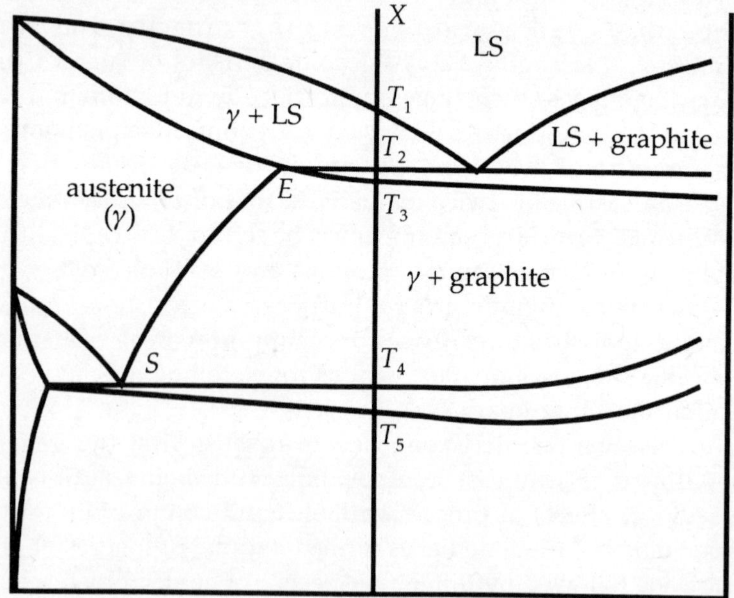

Fig. 4.1: Vertical section of the iron-carbon-silicon ternary alloy system diagram (from AFS The cupola and its operation, 3rd edn., 1965).

(*i*) The eutectic point at 4.30% C is shifted to 3.60% C and the eutectic horizontal becomes a narrow eutectic zone.
(*ii*) The greatest extent of the single phased austenite region is lowered from 2% C to 1.5% C.
(*iii*) The eutectoid point is shifted from 0.80% C to 0.60% C.
(*iv*) The eutectoid horizontal line is changed to the narrow eutectoid zone and the temperature of eutectoid reaction is raised.

Now, the mechanism of solidification of a hypoeutectic gray iron of the composition represented by the vertical line of the above figure can be discussed in detail as follows.

As the liquid iron cools from the pouring temperature, the solidification starts at point T_1 with the formation of primary dendrites of austenite and the amount of the latter increases with further fall of temperature. The carbon contents of these austenites are lower than the liquid from which they are forming and as a result the remaining liquid is enriched in carbon by its precipitation and changes its composition in accordance with the line T_1 C. On further cooling as the temperature approaches the eutectic interval, the remaining liquid approaches the eutectic point C in composition.

The eutectic freezing commences at the point T_2 with the formation of two solids, austenite and graphite in the form of spherical cells between and around the primary austenite dendrites. These cells grow further through cooling in the eutectic temperature range T_2 to T_3 and the graphite is formed as irregular thin crystals (flakes) in a background of austenite in these cells. At point T3, the eutectic freezing is completed and the austenite has the composition with respect to carbon marked by point E.

Further cooling between the point T_3 and T_4, the changes take place in the solid state and the precipitation of carbon in the form of graphite occurs from the austenite whose composition changes in accordance with the line ES. The graphite precipitated in this temperature range does not produce a new flake structure, but is deposited on the flakes formed during eutectic freezing.

As the point S is reached, the eutectoid transformation of austenite takes place between the cooling through the temperature range T_4 to T_5. In this temperature range, the austenite changes into a mixture of graphite and ferrite, ferrite + pearlite or pearlite depending on alloy composition and the cooling rate prevailing.

For example, with most favorable graphitizing conditions, only ferrite and graphite is formed whereas with the less severe graphitizing conditions, ferrite and pearlite or only pearlite is formed along with graphite. On further cooling below T_5 to room temperature, little change in the iron takes place.

The solidification of gray iron of eutectic composition proceeds in the same manner as for the hypoeutectic iron as described above except that the primary dendrites of the austenite are absent and the entire solid as solidification is completed, consists of the eutectic dispersion of austenite and graphite flakes. Cooling and transformation to room temperatures then proceeds as outlined. Hypereutectic irons form graphite as the proeutectic phase and this graphite may appear on the molten iron as kish graphite floating on the surface.

4.3 GRAPHITIZATION AND FACTORS AFFECTING

The iron carbide (Fe_3C), called as cementite is not a stable compound and tends to decompose under favourable conditions in accordance to the following reaction as

$$Fe_3C \rightarrow 2Fe + C$$

The carbon so liberated by the above decomposition is in the form of graphite. The rate of decomposition of the carbide is influenced by a number of factors such as composition of the iron and the cooling rate. High carbon and high silicon in the iron promote rapid decomposition of the carbide or may prevent the formation of the carbide during solidification. Similarly, slow cooling during solidification promotes graphitization or prevent the formation of carbide.

As discussed in the section 4.2, there are the three main stages of graphitization which occur during solidification and cooling of the gray iron in the solid state :

1. Graphitization during solidification
2. Graphitization in the solid state by carbon precipitation
3. Graphitization in the solid state during the eutectoid transformation.

Some graphitization also occurs below the eutectoid transformation range down to about 540° C, although this is of lesser importance unless the time spent at that temperature is very long.

4.3.1 Graphitization During Solidification

The size, shape and distribution of graphite flakes actually develop during the solidification of the gray iron. There are marked differences in the type and size of the graphite flakes formed and they are classified according to the standard type and size charts adopted by the ASTM and AFS. There are some eight sizes of the graphite flakes varying in length from more than 4 inches to less than 1/16 inch (these sizes are given in terms of numbers as 1 to 8) and some five types of the graphite flakes designated by the letters from A to D as shown in the Fig. 4.2. Type A graphite represents the random distribution of flakes (Fig. 4.3a) and is considered as normal type and the most desirable in the small size range of No. 5 to 6. Type D and E are called undercooled graphite and represent the abnormal distribution of graphite flakes which are not desired. E type graphite flakes are dendrically segregated with the preferred orientation (Fig. 4.3b) and are most often encountered in hypoeutectic irons, where the graphite flakes precipitate in the interstices of the primary austenite dendrites. The type D flakes of graphite are of the cellular pattern (Fig. 4.3c) and normally form in the light sections or at the surface of the castings where eutectic solidification is rapid. When the eutectic solidification is suppressed from its normal freezing range, the type of the graphite formed changes from A to types D and E. The type B graphite commonly designated as the rosette distribution is formed in irons of near-eutectic composition that solidify with a greater degree of undercooling than type A and all the above three types are often associated with the formation of massive ferrite in the matrix. The type C graphite is referred to as 'kish graphite' and is characteristic of hypereutectic irons. Thus, in general, a number of factors determine the formation of above different types of the graphite flakes such as the composition, melting practice, rates of solidification and transformation (which are mainly determined by the casting section size) and the final treatment of iron before pouring like inoculation. The effect of the above parameters on graphitization will be discussed in subsequent sections.

4.3.2 Graphitization in the Solid State

At the end of freezing process, a gray iron of 3.60% C and 2.10% Si will contain about 2.0% graphitic carbon and 1.50% of carbon

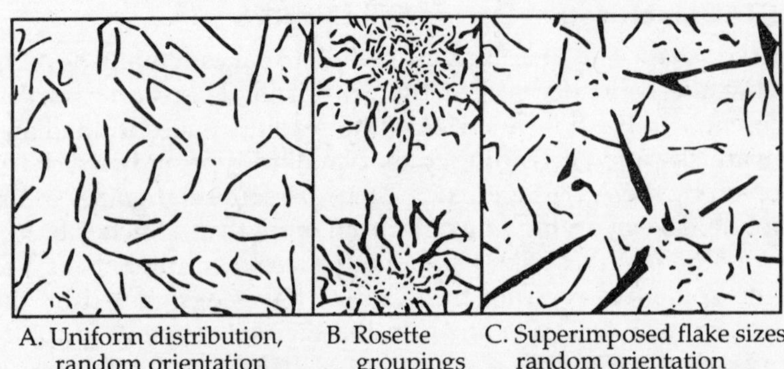

A. Uniform distribution, random orientation

B. Rosette groupings

C. Superimposed flake sizes, random orientation

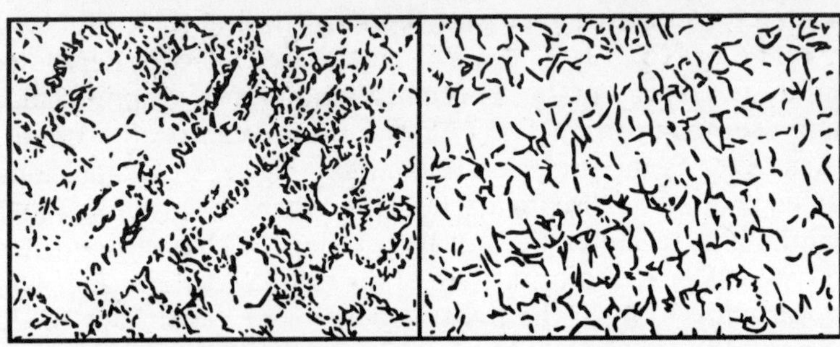

D. Interdendritic segregation, random orientation

E. Interdendritic segregation, preferred orientation

Fig. 4.2: Types of graphite flakes in gray cast irons (From R.W. Heine, C.R. Loper and P.C. Rosenthal, *Principles of Metal Casting*, Tata McGraw Hill, New Delhi, 1976).

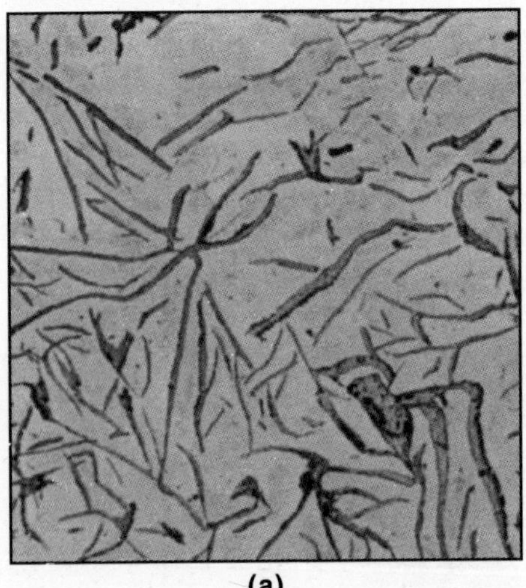

(a)

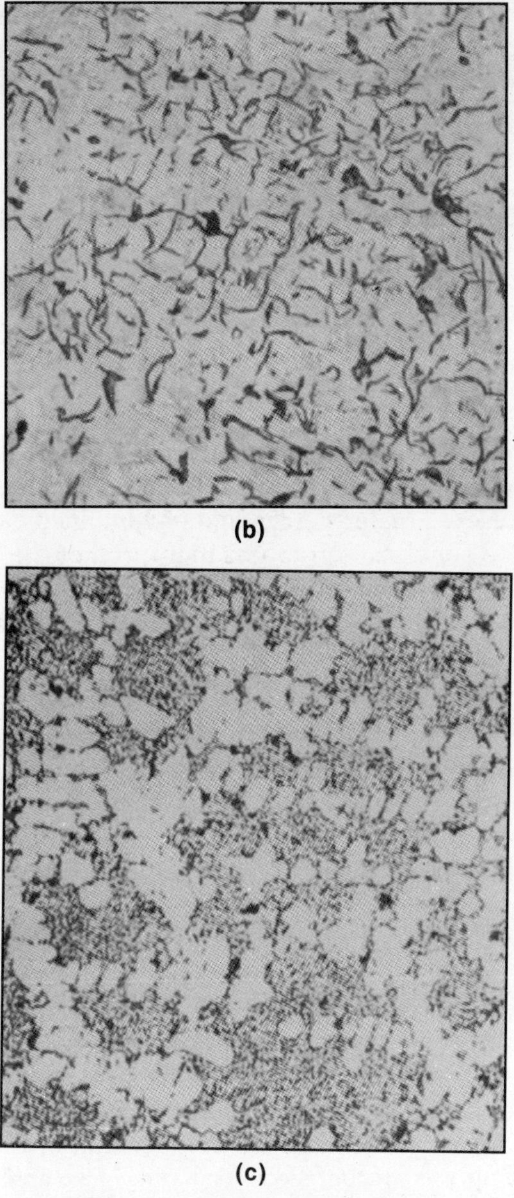

(b)

(c)

Fig. 4.3: Microstructures showing different types of graphite flakes (*a*) Type A graphite flakes, 100X, (*b*) Type E graphite flakes, 100X, (*c*) Type D fine graphite flakes, 200X (From AFS the Cupola and its Operation, 3rd edition, 1965)

dissolved in austenite. Slow cooling promotes precipitation of carbon from the austenite as graphite as the temperature drops to the eutectoid temperature. This carbon rejection is a process of solid-state graphitization and proceeds until about 0.60% C remains in the austenite. The graphite so precipitated joins the previously existing flakes. Very slow cooling through the eutectoid transformation range permits a large portion of the carbon present in the austenite to be rejected as graphite and austenite transforms to ferrite. The iron is then completely graphitized as discussed earlier in the section 4.2. The presence of Mn and S in iron helps in retaining a pearlitic structure or some portion of pearlite even during slow cooling of the casting. Thus gray iron is not completely graphitized and about 0.60% carbon remains in the combined form as cementite (as a constituent of pearlite). However, rapid solid-state cooling and the presence of carbide-forming elements in the iron can cause a greater percentage of combined carbon to be retained. The solid-state graphitization promotes formation of fine graphite flakes regardless of the type. The type D cellular graphite flake, is often intermixed with the ferrite because of the ease with which graphitization may occur.

4.4 INOCULATION OF GRAY CAST IRONS

As mentioned above, one of the factors which has a pronounced effect on formation of types of graphite in gray irons is Inoculation. This treatment of gray iron melt is an important development in gray iron metallurgy to enable to get the most desired structure uniformly despite variations in section thickness of the casting and without appreciably altering its over all chemical composition. Inoculation may be defined as a addition of an element or elements to the molten iron, made primarily for the purpose of controlling microstructure and chilling tendency to a degree not explainable on the basis of composition change of the iron. Thus, inoculation excludes alloy additions made to the molten iron for the sole purpose of affecting the chemical composition of the melt. For example, graphite is a recognized inoculating agent and its addition to the ladle immediately before pouring produces improvement in the microstructure and properties not obtainable by the same increase in carbon content brought about by addition to the cold furnace charge. Late addition is an essential feature of the inoculation process and the effect of inoculation is transient and tends to disappear with the passage of time.

Briefly, inoculation is an important means of controlling chilling tendency and graphite distribution in gray cast irons. The properties of gray irons are very critically affected by metal composition and the cooling rate. The latter perhaps affects the properties of gray cast irons more than in the case of any other metal. In other words, gray iron is very section sensitive. In practice, cooling rates vary not only from casting to casting and from section to section within a casting, but also within a section from the surface in contact with the mould wall to the centre. The inconsistencies in the structure and therefore properties largely arise from the above reasons. The inoculation is a means of reducing section sensitivity of gray irons which enables the foundryman to produce better quality castings and of greater consistency.

The purpose of inoculation is to increase the number of nuclei in the molten iron so that the eutectic solidification, specifically graphitization, can begin with a minimum amount of undercooling. When undercooling is minimized, there is a corresponding reduction in the tendency to form eutectic carbide or white iron, which is referred to as chill. Instead, a more uniform microstructure consisting of small type A graphite flakes is produced. This microstructural change can result in improved machinability and mechanical properties. Inoculation also causes formation of a finer eutectic cell size during freezing which increases the tensile strength of gray irons.

4.4.1 Inoculants Used

In the absence of inoculation, irons tend to undercool and this undercooling is associated with the formation of types D and E graphite. Inoculated irons solidify at a higher temperature. Among the substances employed as inoculating agents are : graphite; certain grades of ferrosilicon containing small amounts of calcium and aluminium, calcium-silicon with calcium in the range of 30 to 35 per cent; and certain complex alloys containing various combinations of aluminium, calcium, zirconium, manganese, titanium, barium and chromium with silicon as a base element. Table 4.1 gives typical analysis of some ladle inoculants used.

TABLE 4.1: TYPICAL ANALYSES OF SOME LADLE INOCULANTS USED[12]

Sl. No.	Inoculant	Composition – Percent								
		C	*Ca*	*Cr*	*Mn*	*Si*	*Ti*	*Zr*	*Al*	*Fe*
1.	Ca-Metal		100							
2.	Ca-Si		30-35			60-65				
3.	Ca-Si-Ti		5-8			45-50	9-11		1.5	Bal.
4.	Cr-Si-Mn-Ti-Ca	3.0	1*	38-42	8-11	14-16	1*		1*	Bal.
5.	Cr-Si-Mn-Ti-Ca	3.0	1*	28-32	14-16	15-21	1*		1*	Bal.
6.	Cr-Si-Mn-Zr (3 grades)			30-52	5-10	14-35		1-6		Bal.
7.	FeSi		0.5-0.8			80-90			1.25*	Bal.
8.	FeSi		0.5-0.8			74-78			1.25*	
9.	Graphite	90-100								
10.	Mo-Si**					30*				
11.	Ni-Si***					30*				Bal.
12.	Si-C	28-46				45-56				
13.	Si-C	50				42*				Bal.
14.	Si-Mn				20-25	47-54		5-7	1.75	
15.	Si-Mn-Zr		2.5		5-7	60-65		5-7	1.75	
16.	Si-Ti					20-25	20-27			
17.	Si-Zr					47-52		35-40		Bal.
18.	Si-Zr					39-43		12-15		Bal.

* Approximate **60% Mo ***60% Ni

Certain inoculants are classified as balanced or stabilizing inoculants as opposed to simple chill reducing inoculants. These stabilizing inoculants contain carbide stabilizing elements such as Cr, Mn, Ti and Zr. Irons treated with these inoculants are less section sensitive and a reduction in chill takes place at edges and in light sections of the castings treated.

4.4.2 Mechanisms of Inoculation

The exact mechanism of inoculation has not yet been determined. However, it has been demonstrated that successful inoculation is accompanied by an increase in the number of eutectic cells formed during eutectic solidification and therefore, a decrease in the eutectic cell size takes place. It is believed that inoculants promote the formation of gray iron by increasing the number of nuclei for eutectic solidification but the mechanism by which they increase melt nucleation is not clearly understood. Investigators have put forward different theories to explain the mechanism of inoculation and most of them are based on a nucleation mechanism. However, upto the present time, no conclusive evidence has been obtained to establish any one theory.

The different theories put forward are[13-16].

1. The Graphite Nuclei Theory
2. Degassification Theory
3. The Silicate-Slime Theory
4. The Undercooling Theory
5. The Carbide Stability Theory
6. Surface Tension or Surface Energy Theory

4.4.2.1 The Graphite Nuclei Theory

According to this theory, graphite particles in the melt act as nuclei to begin the graphitization phenomenon. Inoculation is considered as the addition of effective graphite nuclei to the molten iron. The presence (or increase) of the number of effective nuclei makes the iron more like to form type A graphite at any given cooling rate. This theory is substantiated by the fact that late additions of solid elemental carbon (granular graphite) to an iron normally solidifying with type D or E to change to type A graphite. The presence of silicon in many inoculants showers fine graphite nuclei in the melt due to its powderful graphitizing action. The tendency of superheated irons to form type D and E in preference to type A can be explained by this theory as this high melt superheat leads to destruction of graphite nuclei present in the iron.

4.4.2.2 Degassification Theory

This theory explains the mechanism of inoculation on the basis of reactions occurring between the inoculant and dissolved or chemically combined gases such as O_2, H_2, N_2 etc. These degasification reactions may produce inoculation by the elimination of "chill forming" gases and the formation of the inclusions in the melt which may act as effective nuclei. It is known that inoculated irons show "wearing off (fading) effect" if molten iron is held for an appreciable time between inoculation and pouring. The effect of inoculation gradually fades and even may be eliminated. Thus, the degasification theory holds that this wearing off is due to reabsorption of the gases which were eliminated by the inoculation. It is also a fact that most of the effective inoculants are deoxidizers.

4.4.2.3 The Silicate-Slime Theory

This theory provides for submicroscopic "slime" or "pulp" of ferrous silicate inclusions which act as nuclei for the formation of coarse graphite. This theory is supported by the fact that a slag which removes silicon or ferrous oxide helps to the formation of fine graphite.

4.4.2.4 The Undercooling Theory

This theory is an extension of the nucleation theory which argues that type D and E graphites are formed as a result of undercooling during solidification and that nucleation which results from addition of the inoculating agent prevents this undercooling and produces the durable type A graphite.

4.4.2.5 The Carbide Stability Theory

According to this theory, the changes in carbide stability affect the availability of carbon for flake graphite formation and thereby influence flake size and shape. This theory is supported by the fact that inoculation is accompanied by a reduction in chilling tendency.

4.4.2.6 *Surface Tension or Surface Energy Theory*

According to this, the inoculating agent influences the size and shape of graphite particles by supplying or removing an absorbed substance from the graphite-iron interface thereby promoting the formation of certain graphite forms due to surface energy change.

4.4.3 Fading of Inoculation

As mentioned in one of the theories of inoculation, the effect of inoculation falls off 'wears off' in a relatively short period of time. All the inoculants used suffer from this fading effect though not equally. The present understanding is that the fading is most rapid immediately after making the addition of inoculant to the melt and that it becomes more gradual until the inoculating effect completely disappears after a period of 20 minutes or so. Perhaps, the treated metal is in a superinoculated state just after inoculation.

4.4.4 Techniques of Inoculation

Several methods of inoculation have been developed[12,17,18] with the primary aims of minimizing the fading effect and getting uniform distribution of the inoculant in the molten iron.

4.4.4.1 *Ladle Inoculation*

This is a common technique of treating the molten iron with the inoculating agent before pouring in the mould. The method is to add a small quantity of the inoculant in the range of 0.15 to 0.5% by weight of the melt depending on the potency of the inoculant used. The inoculant is added to the molten iron at the point where the metal stream from the transfer ladle hits the metal in the pouring ladle. A small heel of metal should be allowed to accumulate in the bottom of the ladle before addition is made. This method ensures good mixing action as well as uniform distribution of the inoculant throughout the iron.

4.4.4.2 *Instantaneous Ladle Inoculation*

In another variation of the above method of inoculation, the inoculant is added in the form of a solid bar and the lower end of which rests on the pouring lip of the ladle and dissolves in the stream of the liquid iron throughout the pouring cycle. The physical make up of the rod and pouring temperature of the metal influences in a major way the rate of dissolution of the inoculant in this way. Usually, the time elapsed from inoculation to pouring is 1 to 12 minutes at the inoculation temperature of 1500° C to 1400° C.

4.4.4.3 Stream Inoculation

This method has the advantage in that the inoculant is added late in the production process so that the effect of the time lost in inoculation can be greatly reduced. In this method, the inoculant is added to the stream of metal flowing from the pouring ladle into the mould such that last metal entering the mould is treated similarly to the first metal. A maximum particle size of 8 to 30 mesh and a minimum size of about 100 mesh of the inoculant are recommended for the treatment and the addition levels range from 0.10 to 0.15% of the weight of the melt.

4.4.4.4 Mould Inoculation

It is a novel method of inoculation developed to counteract the fading effect. In this method, the inoculant in the form of fine powder is placed either in the base of the sprue or in a suitable chamber in the runner system of the mould before the metal is poured into the mould. This process works out well but to insure uniform inoculation, alloy solution rate and gating design must be carefully controlled. In another variation of this technique, inoculants in the form of lumps, pellets or briquettes are added in the pouring basin, bases of the sprues or runner systems of the mould to eliminate inconsistent results obtained as in case of using the loose fine powder of the inoculant.

4.4.4.5 Controlled Quality (CQ) Inoculation

In this method, a special steel wire having a core composed of the inoculant is fed directly into the metal stream at a controlled rate while pouring. As the wire melts in the molten metal, the inoculant is thoroughly and uniformly mixed with the metal. Since the metal immediately enters the mould after inoculation, no inoculant fading takes place. A usual amount of the inoculant added is 0.02 to 0.03%. This process of inoculation has the potential of computerized control of the inoculating procedure used which can be used advantageously with automatic moulding and pouring.

4.5 COMPOSITIONS, MICROSTRUCTURES AND PROPERTIES OF GRAY IRONS

The following Table 2 gives the composition range for the different elements present in unalloyed gray cast irons normally produced in commercial practice.

TABLE 4.2: COMPOSITIONS OF COMMERCIAL GRAY CAST IRONS

Elements	%
Carbon	2.60-3.75%
Silicon	1.25-2.75%
Manganese	0.40-0.90%
Sulfur	0.05-0.14%
Phosphorus	0.05-1.00%

All the elements present in gray irons exert some influence on the microstructure of the gray irons obtained.

4.5.1 Effect of Composition on Microstructure

Carbon: Carbon in gray iron can be present from about 2.5 to 4.5% by weight and occurs in two forms, as elemental carbon in the form of graphite and combined carbon as cementite (Fe_3C). The analysis of the iron normally shows the total carbon percentage in the iron. The degree of graphitization can be expressed by the following relationship:

% Total carbon = % Graphitic carbon + % Combined carbon

Naturally, if graphitization is complete, the percentage of total carbon and that of gaphitic carbon will be equal. If about 0.5 to 0.80 per cent of the combined carbon exists in gray iron, the microstructure is then largely pearlitic.

Silicon: It can be present in gray iron from about 1.0 to 3.50% by weight and it is a strong promoter of gaphitization. Low percentages of silicon are not sufficient to cause graphitization during solidification but can cause nucleation and graphitization in the solid state at high temperature (e.g. during heat treatment). Certain silicon percentages will cause limited graphitization during solidification and a mottled iron, partly white and partly gray may form. Increasing carbon and silicon contents in gray iron promotes the appearance of massive ferrite in the microstructure of the iron and thus have a softening and weakening effect on the iron.

Phosphorus: In the presence of phosphorus beyond 0.10% in the iron, an additional constituent appears in the microstructure. This is a phosphorus rich structure known as steadite. Phosphorus concentrates in the remaining liquid during eutectic cell formation and at a certain concentration, steadite appears as the last solid to form in the iron. It is a eutectic type structure consisting of iron with phosphorus in solution and iron phosphide (Fe_3P). With increasing phosphorus in the iron the amount of steadite formed increases.

Carbon Equivalent Value (CEV): Phosphorus increases the effectiveness of carbon and silicon. Therefore, the amount of eutectic graphite formed in the structure of a gray iron depends on its carbon, silicon and phosphorus contents. The effects of these elements are expressed interms of a carbon equivalent value (CEV) where:

$$\text{Carbon equivalent value} = \%\ \text{total carbon} + \%\ \text{silicon}/3 + \%\ \text{phosphorus}/3$$

i.e. the carbon equivalent is the total carbon content plus one-third of the silicon content plus one-third of the phosphorus content. As the carbon equivalent value increases so the amount of graphite in the structure of the iron increases. Irons with CEV < 4.30 are hypoeutectic and irons with CEV > 4.30 are hypereutectic and contains primary graphite in the structure.

Carbon equivalent value (CEV) can not be directly measured but can be calculated from the final analysis of the iron. However, in control testing in the foundry, a Carbon Equivalent Liquidus (CEL) is determined in order to assess metal composition interms of its suitability for use to pour a given grade of iron. The carbon equivalent liquidus (CEL) is determined by the expression as:

$$\text{CEL} = \%\ \text{total carbon} + \%\ \text{silicon}/4 + \%\ \text{phosphorus}/2$$

Sulphur and Manganese: Sulfur is one of the important modifying elements present in gray irons. A low-sulfur iron-silicon-carbon alloy containing sulfur $< 0.01\%$ will graphitize most completely. Higher sulfur percentages favour the retention of a completely pearlitic microstructure in a gray iron and thus it is carbide stabilizing element.

The influence of sulfur should be considered relative to its reaction with the manganese present in the iron. Sulfur alone will form FeS in the iron and this compound segregates into grain boundaries during freezing and precipitates during the final stages of freezing. However, when manganese is present, MnS or complex manganese-iron sulfides are formed depending on Mn content. When MnS is formed, the effect of sulfur in causing a pearlitic microstructure is lost to a great extent. The effect of Mn alone as an alloying element is to resist graphitization. Therefore, Mn above that necessary to react with the sulfur will assist in retaining the pearlitic microstructure.

4.5.2 Effect of Composition and Other Factors on Properties

The microstructure, chemical composition and mechanical properties are intimately related. However, there are many other factors which affect the microstructure and chemical composition variations such as the cooling rate and therefore will also affect the properties.

4.5.2.1 Engineering Properties

Tensile and Transverse Strengths and Hardness: The mechanical properties of a gray cast iron depend mainly on its composition, degree of nucleation of graphite and the cooling rate since all above factors determine the form and amount of graphite and the type of the matrix obtained in its cast structure. The effect of carbon and silicon contents can be expressed in terms of the carbon equivalent value of the iron. As for as the effect of the carbon alone is concerned, increasing its content beyond the amount in combined form results in an increase in the amount of graphite present with a consequent lowering of tensile and transverse strengths. Silicon also acts as a graphitizer but it strengthens and hardens ferrite and in this manner increases the strength of the iron. The combined effect of the above two elements is expressed in terms of CEV which is related to the tensile strength as shown by the following table:

TABLE 4.3: VARIATION OF TENSILE STRENGTH (TS) WITH THE CARBON EQUIVALENT VALUE (CEV) OF GRAY IRONS[19]

Minimum TS values	(in ton/in^2)	10	12	14	17	20	23	26
	(in N/mm^2)	150	180	220	260	300	350	400
Approximate CEV		4.5	4.3	4.1	3.85	3.65	3.5	3.4

It is obvious that strengths of all these grades of gray irons increase as CEV reduces. The tensile strength (TS) is related to the hardness (BHN) of the iron and the TS/BHN ratio is subject to variations due to the influence of various types of flakes of graphite formed. The effects of the type and size of the graphite have been studied and the highest tensile strength at a given hardness is obtained when small A type graphite flake is formed. On the other hand, a poor TS is obtained at a given hardness when type D graphite flake is formed.

The relationship between the hardness and strength of gray iron is not as direct as is the case with steel. In general, the hardness increases with strength. But it is possible to markedly increase TS of the iron by inoculation and at the same time slightly decrease the hardness.

Gray cast irons are also section sensitive as the latter governs the cooling rate. With decrease in section thickness of an iron of a given CEV, the iron becomes progressively harder and stronger. This is because the cooling rate also determines the microstructure formed. Rapid cooling causes increased hardness and tensile strength only so long as it does not produce a white or chilled iron or excessively bad type D graphite structure. Thicker sections (i.e. slow cooling) results in formation of coarse graphite flakes and lamellar pearlite and finally the appearance of ferrite which causes softening and weakening of the gray irons.

Compressive, Tortional and Shear Strengths: In addition to tensile and transverse strengths, there are other strengths of gray irons which deserve specific mention. The compressive strength of gray iron is an outstanding property and has a great significance in applications of this iron. It is three to five times greater than the tensile strength of gray irons. The strength in torsion is about 1.20 to 1.40 times the strength in tension. The shear strength of gray iron is also about 1.0 to 1.60 times its tensile strength.

Yield Strength and Modulus of Elasticity: Gray irons do not exhibit a definite value of yield strength. The modulus of elasticity intension is also variable depending on microstructure of the iron.

Endurance Limit and Ductility: The endurance limit of gray is less sensitive to notches and is about 35 to 50 per cent of its tensile strength. However, gray iron is a brittle material and its percent elongation is less than one per cent.

Wear Resistance: It is another outstanding property of gray iron which is exemplified in its use for many applications such as piston rings, cylinder liners, crank shafts, clutch plates, bake drums, gears and engine blocks.

Machinability: Gray iron is among the most readily machinable ferrous alloys. The best machinability is obtained in the softer irons. Most gray irons have a hardness range of 130 to 240 BHN and a combination of moderate strength and hardness gives good machinability.

Damping Capacity : It is an ability of a material to absorb energy due to vibrations and thus dampen the vibrations. Gray irons super seed the plain carbon steels in this respect. This property of gray irons makes smooth operations of internal-combustion engines or other structures such as lathe machines where vibrations occur in operation of such machines.

Heat and Corrosion Resistance: The heat resistance of gray irons is the ability to resist scaling and retain moderate strength at elevated temperatures. It is a desirable property in many applications of gray irons such as furnace parts, melting pots, gas burners etc. It can be further improved by alloying gray irons. Like heat resistance, the corrosion resistance of gray irons is important in some applications like water mains and other pipe applications.

Electrical Resistance and Heat Treatable Ability: The electrical resistance of gray irons is sufficiently high so that they are used extensively for resistance grids. Gray irons are also readily heat treatable and can be hardened and tempered like steels to improve many properties for use in several applications.

4.5.2.2 Foundry Properties

For several reasons, gray irons are among the most easily cast of all ferrous alloys such as their low melting points, good fluidity and low shrinkage characteristics. Gray irons have above such foundry properties to an optimum degree.

Fluidity Characteristics: Gray irons are the most fluid ferrous casting alloys. Very intricate and thin sections of complex castings may be produced. Fluidity of gray irons is expressed interms of lengths of a standard fluidity spiral casting and is related to composition and pouring temperature by the formula :

$$\text{Fluidity (inches)} = 14.9 \times \text{CEL} + 0.05T - 155$$

where $\text{CEL} = \%C + \frac{1}{4} \times \%Si + \frac{1}{2} \times \%P$

and T = Pouring Temperature in °F.

The most fluid iron has approximately the eutectic composition (CEL of 4.55). The fluidity increases as the pouring temperature increases. However, the hypereutectic gray irons suffer an extreme loss of fluidity due to kishing, i.e., the precipitation of graphite flakes as the liquid metal cools. Besides the carbon, silicon and phosphorus, other elements present in iron such as sulfur may also influence the fluidity of gray irons.

Wide Pouring Temperature Range: High fluidity of gray irons is also due to the fact that they have low melting point and can be superheated to much above their melting point without any damage. They can be poured with 50°C to as high as 350°C melt superheat. This wide working temperature range permits ease of manipulation in the foundry, reladling and adequate time for pouring.

Low Shrinkage Characteristics: Gray irons have low value of total shrinkage due to their favourable freezing characteristics (graphitization during freezing) and it is often possible to use metal present in runners and gates to be sufficient for feeding the casting without the need of a riser. The use of top gating with its advantage of additional fluid pressure and favourable temperature gradient can be employed for feeding shrinkage of some gray iron castings. In many cases, little or no risering is needed if the mould used is strong.

High Casting Yield: Because little or no risering required, the yield percentage of gray iron castings is high compared with the castings of other ferrous alloys. A yield of 60 to 75% or even higher may be obtained in some gray iron castings.

4.6 GRAY IRON FOUNDRY PRACTICE

4.6.1 Moulding and Casting Practice

Gray iron castings are produced by almost all processes of casting available such as sand casting, permanent mould casting, centrifugal casting etc. Among the sand casting processes, green sand moulding, dry sand moulding core sand moulding, shell moulding, CO_2 sand moulding and high pressure sand moulding are adopted. Out of these sand casting processes, green sand moulding is most commonly used for production of gray iron castings.

The moulding sand mixtures used should have sufficient clay to provide high compression and shear strength and should be able to absorb sand expansion. It should also have sufficient moisture to activate the binder and provide requisite good permeability. Both sodium base and calcium base bentonites or their combination are used as the bonding material. Additives like sea coal, coke, graphite, pitch etc. may be used in sand mixtures for producing a reducing atmosphere in the mould for preventing oxidation of the metal and other sand reactions and also to provide better surface finish (when used in the form of mould coatings). Use of wood, cereals, oat hulls etc. is made along with sea coal to accommodate sand expansion and provide better stripping characteristics. Both new and system sands are used as the base material of sand mixtures. The amount of sea coal used varies depending upon the size of casting. For example, it may vary from 1% for small castings to 10% for heavy casting.

The following may be typical green sand mixtures used with the properties:

Silica sand of AFS grain fineness number	: 60 to 75
Clay content	: 6 to 8%
Moisture content	: 3.5 to 4%
Volatile combustible matter	: 5 to 6%
Green compression strength	: 1.2 to 1.35 kg/cm^2
Permeability	: 80 to 100

Gray iron expands during eutectic solidification because of formation of graphite and this is most pronounced in higher carbon equivalent irons, in which more graphite is precipitated. This expansion stresses the moulding material, causes an enlargement of the mould cavity if the mould is not sufficiently compacted. This phenomena is known as 'Mould Wall Movement' and can lead to formation of shrinkage defects. Such mould wall movement due to weak green sand moulds may be prevented by ramming the sand mixtures to a sand hardness number of 90 to 93. To produce hallow castings, cores of different types such as oil sand cores, CO_2 sand cores, hot box sand, cold set sands etc. are used.

Dry sand moulding, CO_2 sand moulding and shell moulding are adopted where greater strength and better permeability of the moulds are required and good surface finish is desired.

The permanent mould casting is employed for producing small sized gray iron castings weighing less than 15 kg. This process is suitable for production of pressure castings (e.g. castings for compressors and hydraulic cylinders). Generally, hypereutectic iron compositions are employed to obtain high fluidity.

In centrifugal casting of gray irons, usually horizontal axis casting machines are employed for making cast iron pipes for transport of water and gas.

4.6.2 Melting and Pouring

The melting furnaces used for melting of gray irons have been discussed in detail in Chapter 2 and 3. Besides cupolas, air or rotary furnaces, electric arc and induction furnaces are used for melting of gray irons. The latter are used where high grade irons of precise chemical control and with a high degree of superheat are required. Duplex melting practice is also adopted. Normally, a pouring temperature range of 1260 to 1450°C is employed depending upon the composition, section thickness and size of the casting poured.

4.6.3 Gating and Risering

The gating and risering practice used for gray iron castings is less critical than for other metals. Gates used for gray iron castings are usually 50 to 80% smaller than those required for steels, Cu and Al alloys. The gating is designed to allow entry of the metal at velocities fast enough to prevent misruns and cold shut defects. Slag and dirt traps are commonly used to introduce clean metal into the mould. An optimum pouring rate is desired to produce quality castings. Mildly pressurized gating ratios of the order of 1 : 2 : 1, 1 : 2 : 05, 1 : 4 : 1 and 2 : 7 : 1 etc. are commonly adopted. A non-pressurized gating system with gating ratio of 1:4:3 may be also adopted for certain castings which helps in displacing non-metallic inclusions into the runner extension and minimizing spurting of the metal from the gate into the mould cavity. Gates should be also located in such away that directional solidification is promoted.

Little or no risering is needed for the purpose of feeding shrinkage of gray iron castings as discussed under the shrinkage characteristics of such irons. Sometimes, use of proper runner can solve the purpose of feeding the casting. However, risering is very critical for other requirement of riser such as mould wall movement, which occurs in case of weak sand moulds used for gray iron castings. In such cases, stronger moulds are prepared and careful risering is needed. The riser should be located in areas of the casting section which are last to solidify. Side risers are found to be more effective than top risers in such cases.

4.6.4 Cleaning of Castings

This includes all operations necessary to the removal of sand, scale and excess metal from the casting. The casting is separated from the moulding sand after it has solidified and transported to the cleaning department. The burned-on sand and scale are removed to improve the surface appearance of the casting and the excess metal, in the form of fins, wires, gates and risers etc. is cut off. Other various cleaning operations are carried out by blasting, tumbling, chipping, grinding etc. Defective castings may be salvaged by welding or other repairs. After inspection and testing of the casting, it is ready for shipment or further processing such as heat treatment, surface treatment or machining. In certain cases, metallic, ceramic or organic coatings may be applied which extend the range of usefulness of the gray iron castings.

4.7 HEAT TREATMENT OF GRAY IRON CASTINGS

Although most gray iron castings are used in the as-cast condition, heat treatment is employed in certain cases to meet the specific requirements of the casting. The most commonly used methods of heat treatment are annealing, stress relieving and normalizing. However, other standard heat treatments such as quenching and tempering, austempering and martempering are also used on limited occasions. Gray irons can be also flame or induction hardened depending on requirement.

4.7.1 Annealing

There are three principal processes of annealing used for gray iron castings depending on the composition and section thickness employed. They are employed primarily for the purpose of improving machinability and therefore, all the three heat treatments involve the production of a ferritic matrix.

4.7.1.1 Ferritizing or Subcritical Anneal

It consists of heating the casting to a temperature of 700 to 760° C or just below the eutectoid transformation temperature and holding it for a period of one hour per inch of the casting section thickness. The casting is then cooled at the rate of not more than 100° C per hour to avoid retention of cooling stresses. There is reduction in strength and hardness of the casting with improvement in the machinability as a result of this treatment.

4.7.1.2 Medium or Full Annealing

This treatment is applied to the castings when the above heat treatment is unable to convert the iron into a ferritic matrix because of the presence of alloying elements or minor amount of the chill. In this process, the casting is heated to a higher temperature of 800 to 900° C (i.e. above the eutectoid transformation temperature) and soaked at this temperature for a period of one hour per inch of the section thickness of the casting and then slowly cooled through the eutectoid transformation range. The casting is then air cooled after a temperature of 675° C is reached.

4.7.1.3 Graphitizing Anneal

This is the third form of the annealing treatment used in case of gray iron castings to remove presence of massive carbides or severe chilling. It consists of heating the casting to a temperature of 900 to 925° C for a short period and then slowly cooling in a furnace or air cooling through the eutectoid transformation range depending upon whether a ferritic matrix or pearlitic matrix is desired.

4.7.2 Normalizing

In this process, castings are heated to a temperature of 875 to 900°C and held for about one hour per inch of the section thickness followed by air cooling to form a pearlitic matrix.

4.7.3 Hardening and Tempering

Such heat treatment may be employed to obtain increased wear resistance in gray irons. It consists in heating the iron to 850 to 925C, holding for 20 to 30 minutes at this temperature and then quenching into oil or water to produce a martensitic structure. The quenched iron may then be tempered at various temperatures to reduce the hardness as desired. Such treatments may be applied to cylinder liners, gears, cams, rollers etc. to obtain the improved wear resistance.

The flame or induction hardening of the wearing surfaces may be more desirable than quenching and tempering the entire casting as many castings are likely to crack when quenched from high temperature

4.7.4 Stress Relieving

It is used for the purpose of relieving stresses induced in the casting during solidification. The process consists of heating the casting to a temperature of 500 to 650° C depending on composition, holding at this temperature for 2 to 8 hours and air cooling.

White and Malleable Irons and Foundry Practice

5.1 INTRODUCTION

White cast iron is an iron which contains no free carbon and a substantial portion of the carbon present is combined with iron to form a compound known as iron carbide (Fe_3C) or cementite. The latter is a very hard and brittle substance (having hardness > 750 BHN) and its presence as a part of the structure of white iron accounts for the hardness, brittleness and abrasion resistance of this iron. Due to the absence of graphite and the presence of light etching massive cementite, the fracture of white iron is white and lustrous in appearance as opposed to the dark fracture of gray iron. Since this iron is hard and unmachinable, it has less extensive direct application than the other forms of iron. White iron castings are used for applications involving wear resistance such as bearings and spacer tools in farm machinary, tumbling and pulverizing mill liners, ore crushing plants, hammers and parts of ceramic industry. The chilled cast irons which have white iron structures at the surface are used in applications where abrassive wear resistance on wearing surfaces are desired such as rail road freight car wheels, grain mill rolls and rolls for crushing ores and rolling metals. The main application of white irons is in the manufacture of malleable irons.

Malleable cast iron may be defined as a ductile ferrous alloy produced by the heat treatment of white cast iron. It has a microstructure consisting of compacted inclusions of graphite, called temper carbon nodules, in a matrix of ferrite or pearlite or some other decomposition product of austenite. This form of graphitic carbon interrupts the matrix to a minimum degree and results in a alloy which is highly machinable and at the same time is sufficiently tough and ductile. In fact, the malleable iron is the most readily machinable ferrous alloy which combines good ductility and toughness with adequate strength and has corrosion resistance for certain applications, magnetic properties and uniformity resulting from 100 per cent heat treatment of all castings produced. The malleable iron castings find an extensive application which reflects a need for one or more of the fore-going properties. The principal users of the malleable castings are the automotive and truck industries, producers of construction machineries and agricultural equipment makers.

Malleable irons are hypoeutectic in composition and the production of white cast iron is the first and an essential step in the manufacture of malleable iron. It is therefore a necessity to discuss first the mechanism of solidification and transformation of white iron which is a fundamental of the metallurgy of malleable irons.

5.2 SOLIDIFICATION OF A WHITE CAST IRON

The formation of iron carbide in white cast irons is a case of metastable equilibrium as the carbide phase is not a stable phase like graphite. Its formation is favoured by low carbon and silicon contents, by fast cooling or by both of these parameters. As such, an iron-iron carbide (Fe-Fe_3C) metastable phase diagram will be relevant for the discussion of the origin of structures formed during freezing of a white cast-iron. Fig. 5.1 represents a simplified schematic diagram of such a metastable Fe-C-Si system presenting the essential features. With reference to this diagram, the freezing and cooling of a hypoeutectic alloy represented by the vertical line marked by the composition A may be described as follows.

As the alloy is cooled from the pouring temperature to point 1, it is in the molten state and at this point during further cooling solid austenite dendrites begin to form and grow until the temperature at point 2 is reached. During above freezing as more and more of austenite forms, the liquid iron is enriched in its solute contents continuously. At point 2, the liquid is of eutectic composition and eutectic freezing begins with further decrease in temperature over a narrow temperature range. The eutectic mixture consisting of two solids, austenite and cementite (usually called as "ledeburite") forms as a result of the eutectic reaction in the spaces between the austenite dendrites. During the eutectic freezing, secondary crystals of austenite (in distinguishable from the primary austenite) and "massive" carbides precipitate until the iron has been completely solidified.

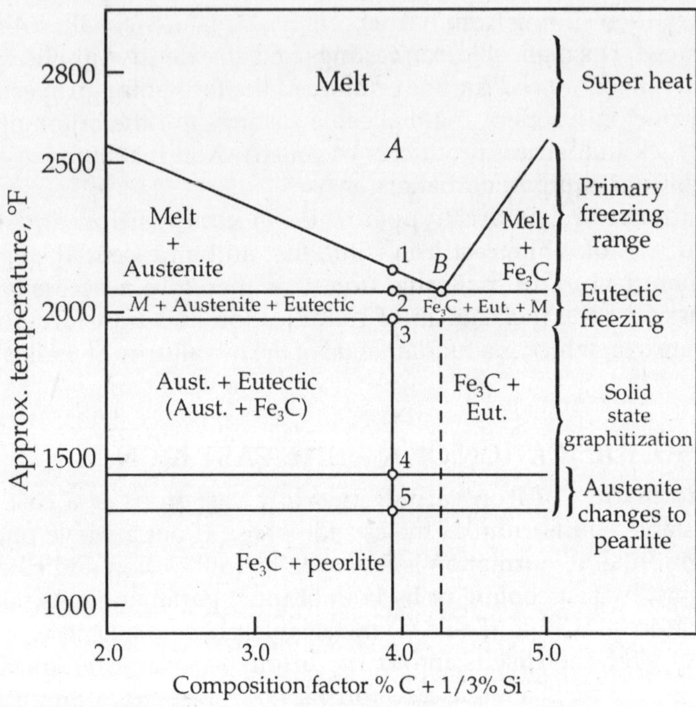

Fig. 5.1: Simplified schematic diagram of a metastable Fe-C-Si system

Further cooling between points 3 and 4 results in the precipitation of carbon from the austenite as carbide since the austenite may contain as much as 2% C at the end of eutectic freezing and when point 4 is reached during further cooling, it may contain about 0.6 to 0.8% C. Between points 4 and 5, the final structural change occurs in the solid state during cooling. The austenite transforms to pearlite (consisting of alternate plates of ferrite and cementite) as a result of the eutectoid reaction over the temperature range of points 4 and 5. The microstructure now consists of relatively large or massive crystals of cementite and pearlite. In cooling from the eutectoid temperature to ambient temperature, the only change is a slight increase in the amount of cementite by precipitation from the ferrite solid solution. Now, both the primary and eutectic crystals of austenite have transformed to pearlite and two types of the cementite crystals are present in the microstructure (Fig. 5.2). These are the large or massive crystals which formed as one constituent of the eutectic solid mixture and the small or lamellar crystals which formed as a part of the pearlite during the eutectoid reaction.

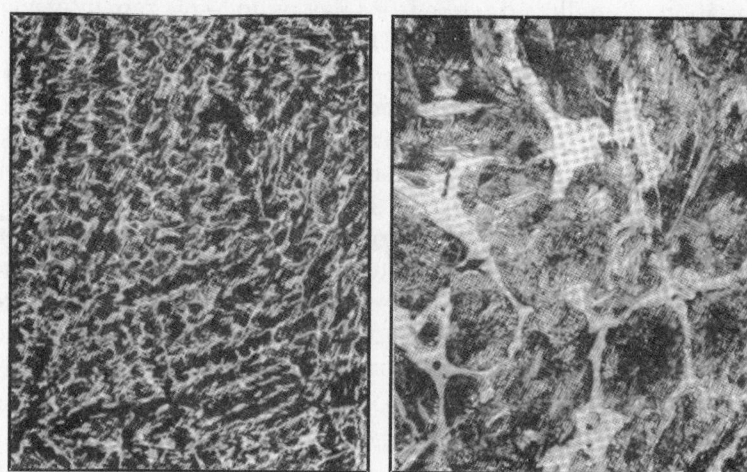

Fig. 5.2: Typical microstructure of etched white iron at low magnification (100X, left) and at high magnification (500X, right) (From Malleable Iron Casting, Malleable Founders Society, Cleveland, Ohio, 1960, p. 337).

In the case of solidification of an alloy of eutectic composition, no precipitation of primary dendrites of austenite occurs and the entire mass of liquid solidifies as the eutectic structure, ledeburite. As cooling further takes place, the transformation takes place in the same manner as described in the case of hypoeutectic iron with the final structure consisting again of massive cementite and pearlite.

Irons of hypereutectic composition solidify with the formation of primary iron carbide (cementite) and this precipitation is followed by the transformation of the remaining liquid to ledeburite as the eutectic freezing takes place. Increasing the carbon content of the white iron increases the hardness of the iron as a result of formation of increased massive cementite which accounts for the high compression strength and abrasion resistance of white irons.

5.3 MICROSTRUCTURES, COMPOSITONS AND PROPERTIES OF WHITE CAST IRONS

As obvious from the above discussion of solidification mechanism of white cast irons, the main factors controlling their microstructures so as to retain carbon in the combined form as cementite are the composition and the cooling rate. In general, low silicon content and rapid cooling rate during freezing promote formation of unalloyed white irons having massive cementates in the matrix of pearlite (Fig. 5.2). The cooling rate can be enhanced by choosing thin section casting or casting against or in metallic moulds. The latter are used to produce chilled cast irons having white iron structures in the surface regions of castings. White cast irons are also made by pouring metal of suitable composition in sand moulds. As mentioned in the earlier section, by increasing the carbon content the proportion of the massive cementite can be increased in the as-cast structure of white cast irons. The presence of such large size cementite particles increases the hardness of the white irons. The latter can be further increased by alloying with nickel, chromium or manganese.

5.3.1 Composition and Engineering Properties

The composition of white iron should be carefully selected in relation to the section thickness of the casting to ensure that the amount of the metal involved can be chilled rapidly enough to produce a white iron structure throughout the casting made. The following give the range of composition selected and the mechanical properties of unalloyed white iron castings:

		%
Carbon	–	1.8 to 3.6
Silicon	–	0.5 to 1.9
Manganese	–	0.25 to 0.80
Sulfur	–	0.05 to 0.20
Phosphorus	–	0.05 to 0.18
Tensile strength (131 to 483 N/mm^2)	–	20,000 to 70,000 psi
Yield strength	–	similar to gray irons
Elongation	–	< 1%
Hardness	–	350 to 600 BHN
Compression strength (1310 to 1638 N/mm^2)	–	200 to 250,000 psi

The hardness of the white cast irons is particularly dependent upon the amount of carbide present although the presence of pearlite matrix does contribute to the total hardness of the white iron. The high carbon white irons are harder than the low carbon irons but are weaker and somewhat more brittle. The high hardness of white cast irons combined with high compression strength makes these irons quite suitable for applications where high wear or abrasion resistance is required.

5.3.2 Foundry Characteristics

The casting properties which affect manufacture of white iron castings are fluidity, shrinkage and feeding characteristics, hot tearing tendency and pouring temperature.

Fluidity: The fluidity of white iron is mainly governed by their composition and temperature of pouring. With increase in the carbon equivalent of the white iron the fluidity increases linearly. The increase in pouring temperature also increases the fluidity. Some changes in fluidity are caused by the melting practice and other variables, but they are secondary to the major effects caused by the composition and temperature. Small white iron castings of 1/16 inches or less in section thickness can be cast if the iron is high in carbon or silicon and poured at high temperature.

Shrinkage and Feeding Characteristics: The white iron has a relatively large solidification shrinkage of the order of 3 to 6 per cent which is reflected by the lower yield percentage of its castings (about 50 per cent). It is difficult to feed the solidification shrinkage of white iron as it solidifies in two stages : firstly, during formation of primary austenite and secondly, during eutectic freezing. The formation of interlocking dendrites of austenite during early stage of freezing makes it difficult for the molten metal to pass from a riser to the casting. As a result, unfed shrinkage leads to formation of cavities with a dendritic pattern. Chills are therefore frequently employed to improve feeding by causing sharp temperature gradients in the casting. Use of chills causes rapid solidification in locations which would not be reached from a riser if normal temperature gradients existed. Usually short feeding distances from the riser to the casting are preferred. Special cares are taken, particularly in feeding of heavy sections isolated by thinner sections.

Hot Tearing: Such high temperature defects may occur in white iron castings during the later stages of freezing i.e. eutectic freezing. Such defects usually occur in locations of extra mass i.e. hot spots. A number of factors affect formation of hot tears in white iron castings such as casting design, gating design, composition of iron and pouring temperature and therefore a number of tricks are required to be used to cope with it. Use of soft and collapsible cores, chills and cracking strips etc. are useful. The strips are thin metal fins attached to the casting over the area where tearing is likely to take place. The fin freezes quickly, extracts heat and helps to hold together the iron when it might rupture.

Pouring Temperature: The pouring temperature of the white iron is generally between 1425 to 1540°C which is substantially higher than gray cast irons which may be poured down to 1260°C. This means that moulding and core sands used must be more heat resistant. As such, synthetic moulding and core sands are preferred.

5.4 TYPES AND COMPOSITIONS OF MALLEABLE IRONS

Essentially, there are two types of malleable irons, namely Ferritic or Standard Malleable Irons and Pearlitic Malleable Irons. As the names suggest, ferritic malleable iron has a ferrite matrix in which compacted inclusions of graphite, called temper carbon nodules are distributed (Fig. 5.3). On the other hand, pearlitic malleable iron has a matrix of pearlite, pearlite + ferrite, tempered martensite or spheroidal carbide (i.e. those containing 0.3 to 0.9% combined carbon in the matrix) along with the interspered nodules of temper carbon (Fig. 5.4). Such irons have superior strength and hardness as a result of the hardening effect of the carbide particles dispersed in the ferrite.

In commercial practice, the term malleable iron refers to the ferritic material. There are two types of ferritic malleable irons, "Blackheart" and "White heart" and these names are derived from the colour of the fracture of the annealed material. The Black heart malleable iron has a matrix of ferrite with interspered nodules of temper carbon. The white heart malleable iron has a different form of the temper carbon and usually contains some combined carbon, because of its composition and method of manufacture.

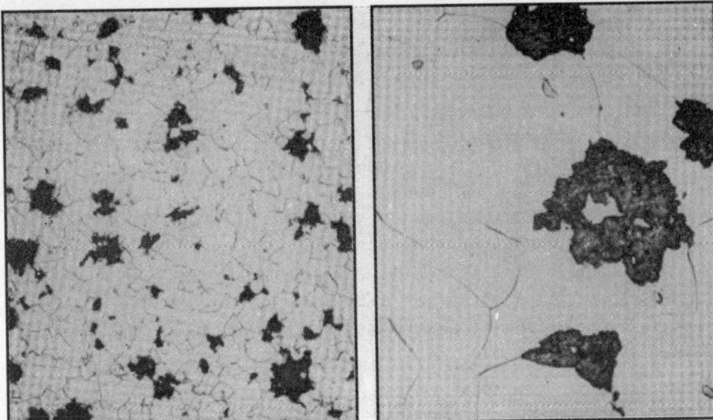

Fig. 5.3: Ferritic malleable iron exhibiting two major constituents, ferrite and temper carbon in the microstructures (at low magnification, 100X left and at high magnification, 500X right) (From Malleable Iron Casting, Malleable Founders Society, Cleveland, Ohio, 1960, p. 337).

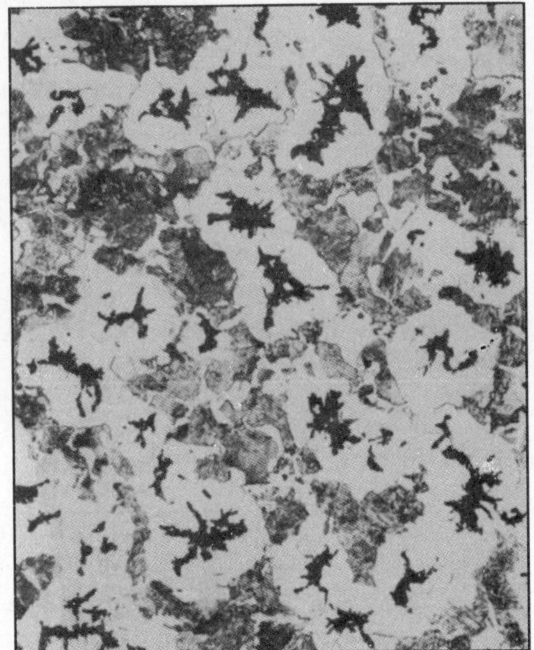

Fig. 5.4: Microstructure of pearlitic malleable iron showing temper carbon nodules in the matrix of ferrite and pearlite (Bull's eye structure) (From Cupola and its Operation, AFS, Illinois, 1965, p. 316).

The term 'Cupola Malleable Iron' is a black heart malleable iron (a ferritic grade material) produced by cupola melting for applications as pipe fittings and similar thin sectioned castings. Such iron has lower strength and ductility and is not usually specified for structural applications.

All the above types of malleable irons, should be completely white and free from graphitic carbon in the as-cast condition when fractured regardless of section size and thickness. The average chemical compositions of the above different types of malleable irons are given in the Table 5.1.

TABLE 5.1: AVERAGE COMPOSITIONS OF DIFFERENT FERRITIC AND PEARLITIC MALLEABLE IRONS[20]

Type of Malleable Iron	%C	%Si	%Mn	%S	%P
White Heart Malleable Iron	2.9-3.4	0.8-0.5	0.2-0.4	0.20	0.10
Black Heart Malleable Iron	2.3-2.6	1.5-1.0	0.3-0.5	0.15	0.10
Cupola Malleable Iron	2.80-3.30	1.10-0.60	0.65	0.25	0.20
Pearlitic Malleable Iron	2.0-2.65	1.65-0.90	0.25-1.25	0.18	0.18

Apart from the above grades of malleable iron, there is also a grade of Alloyed Malleable Iron[21], also called "Special Malleable" as used for special applications. Except the additions of some alloying elements, rest all manufacturing process used for these irons is the same as that used for the ferritic or standard malleable irons. The special properties of these irons are due to the effect of the alloying addition on the matrix of the castings which is usually ferritic.

There are two main kinds of alloyed malleable irons : (1) copper-alloyed malleable iron, and (2) copper-molybdenum-alloyed malleable iron. The former type contains 0.25 to 1.25% Cu which increases resistance to atmospheric corrosion, particularly in sulfurous atmospheres[21]. The second type, alloyed with Cu and Mo, gives extra high strength with no appreciable reduction inductility. In addition to 0.5 to 1.25 per cent of copper, molybdenum is added upto 0.5% to the iron to increase its tensile and yield strengths due to its carbide stabilizing effect.

5.5 THE MALLEABLIZING PROCESS

The annealing heat treatment of the white iron castings used in the manufacture of malleable irons is often called Malleablization. As taken from the mould and cleaned, the as-cast malleable castings are hard and brittle and have a microstructure which contains massive cementite in a pearlitic matrix and is free of graphite. This structure is converted to a soft ductile structure containing temper carbon nodules in the malleablizing process.

The annealing heat treatment used is accomplished in both the batch and continuous furnaces. In the batch process, castings are packed in sealed pots or boxes and surrounded by a supporting packing material such as sand, gravel or mill scale. The containers are stacked in oil, coal or gas fired periodic furnaces subjected to extended annealing cycles for long periods of upto ten days. The sealing in boxes is necessary to avoid undue oxidation, scaling and decarburization.

More modern annealing practice utilizes electric or radiant tube and gas fired continuous furnaces with controlled atmospheres. The latter allows stacking the castings in open baskets and shortens the annealing cycle by permitting more rapid temperature changes. The annealing time in such type of equipment requires from 36 to 72 hours.

5.5.1 Ferritic Malleable Irons

For production of ferritic malleable irons, two types of malleablizing processes are used namely Black heart Process and White Heart Process.

5.5.1.1 Blackheart Process

It is an American Process developed by Seth Boyden in 1826 and is used for production of black heart malleable irons. In this process, white iron castings of suitable chemical compositions are annealed by controlled heating in an inert atmosphere in two stages known as First Stage Graphitization (FSG) and Second Stage Graphitization (SSG). FSG is carried out at about 920 to 950° C and SSG at about 700° C. The annealing is done by controlled heating upto 950°C and maintaining the casting at this temperature for a prolonged period followed by rapid cooling to 700° C. Thereafter, controlled cooling through the critical temperature range promotes secondary graphitization and development of a largely ferritic structure containing temper carbon in the matrix of ferrite with uniform properties from surface to the centre of the casting. The time-temperature cycle used depends on the composition of the iron, the section thickness of the casting and the properties required. A typical time-temperature cycle for a continuous such heat treatment in neutral atmosphere is shown in Fig. 5.5. The casting is slowly heated to the annealing temperature to minimize the risk of cracking and to introduce a large number of graphite nuclei (known as nucleation of graphite). Rapid heating to such temperature will provide fewer graphite nuclei and will increase the time for graphitization. During FSG, sufficient time is allowed for all the eutectic cementite to decompose to austenite + graphite. When this is complete, the casting is cooled relatively quickly to about 750° C and then cooled very slowly through the eutectoid range down to 650° C. This slow cooling during SSG avoids the formation of stable pearlite and allows the austenite to transform to ferrite and graphite. The new graphite so formed deposits on the first stage graphite aggregates. The final structure after cooling therefore consists of graphite aggregates (temper carbon nodules) in a matrix of equiaxed ferrite (Fig. 5.6). The fracture of this structure appears black or sooty due to the presence of the graphite aggregates, and hence such malleable irons are called Black heart.

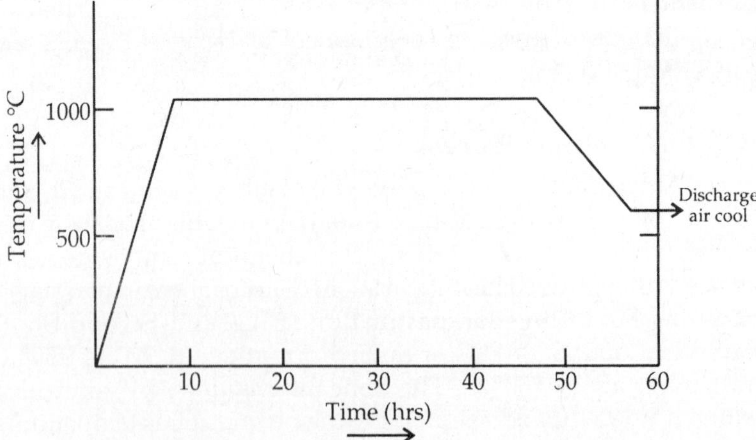

Fig. 5.5: Typical Time-Temperature cycle of a continuous Black heart Process[22]

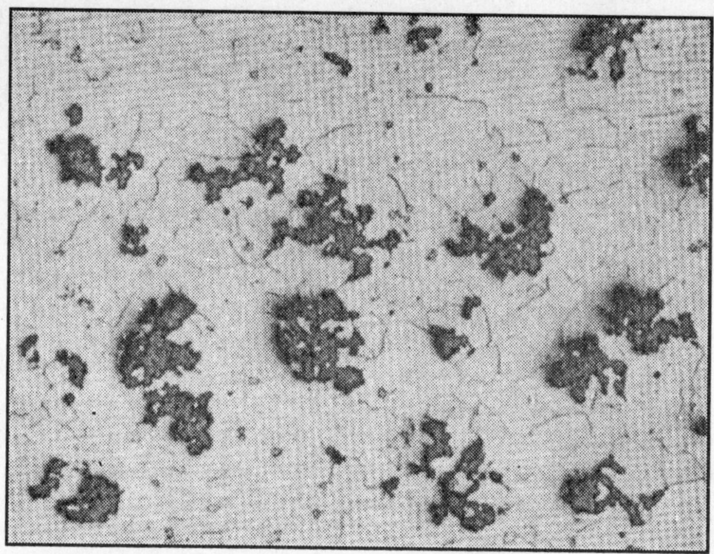

Fig. 5.6: Microstructure of a Black heart malleable iron, X150 (Courtesy of Portcullis Press, Redhill).

The original blackheart process involved pack annealing in sealed cans with inert material and required long total times upto several days. However, shorter batch processes have been developed using controlled atmospheres in bell type or elevator type furnaces with treatment times reduced to 50-70 hours. For large quantity production, continuous furnaces have replaced batch units using nitrogen atmospheres and treatment times from 28 hours to less than 24 hours. Annealing times are shorter in thinner sectioned castings and when silicon contents are as high as possible.

5.5.1.2 White Heart Process

It is a European Process developed by R.A.F. Reaumur in 1722 in which the white iron castings are annealed in a decarburizing atmosphere in order to eliminate as much carbon as possible from surface layers of the castings by oxidation. The result is a material with a soft and ductile skin merging into a high carbon centre, the structure of which consists of nodules or spheroids in a pearlitic or steel like matrix. The decarburization is brought about by oxygen either from air or iron ore coming in contact with the casting at high temperature. The castings are annealed at 950-1050° C. On heating the casting, the as-cast pearlite transforms to austenite so that on reaching the annealing temperature, the structure contains austenite and eutectic cementite. On holding at this temperature, dissolved carbon in the austenite is continually removed from the surfaces of the casting by the decarburizing atmosphere. Simultaneously, the cementite slowly transforms to austenite and graphite. Thin sections of the casting tend to be completely decarburized so that after cooling their structure is similar to that of a mild steel. In thicker sections, there will be a carbon concentration gradient from the edge to centre regions so that after cooling the edges become fully ferritic but the core is pearlitic and may contain graphite aggregates as shown in diagram form in Fig. 5.7. The pearlite in the central regions gives rise to the characteristic white fracture appearance in the test specimens and hence the name White heart is given to these irons.

The extent of the decarburization in a Whiteheart iron depends on manganese to sulfur ratio as well as on section thickness. In an iron with a balanced composition, the structure will be as sketched in Fig. 5.7. However, in an iron with excess sulfur i.e. with a small manganese to sulfur ratio, decarburization is generally more pronounced since graphitization is retarded. Any temper carbon present in the high sulfur iron tends to form nodular shapes.

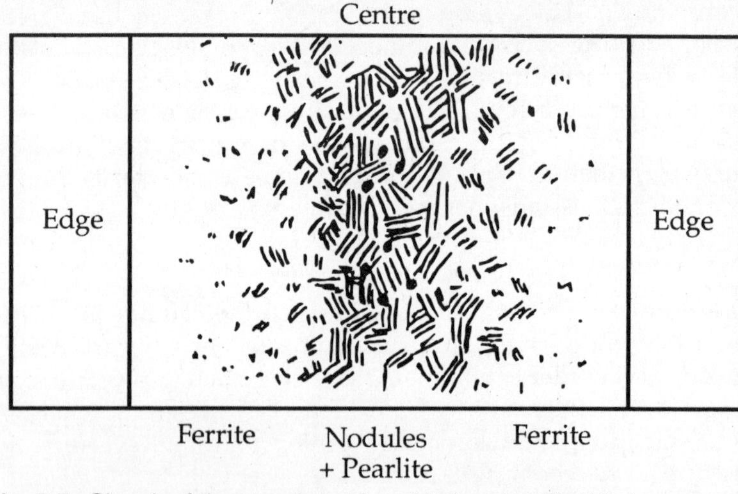

Fig. 5.7: Sketch of the structure of a whiteheart malleable iron across a casting section after heat treatment

In the original white heart process, the castings are packed into heat resistant annealing cans with a mixture of new and used iron oxide ore which is used to generate a decarburizing atmosphere. The loaded cans are sealed and are stacked into batch type furnaces. They are slowly heated to 1000° C and held for about 4 days and then slowly cooled so that the total treatment time can be upto 7 days. However, this pack annealing process is time consuming and can give rise to surface defects due to ore-casting surface reactions. Such defects can be avoided and considerable time can be saved by the use of controlled atmosphere furnaces. In this technique, packing is not necessary as a decarburizing furnace atmosphere is maintained in contact with the casting. A typical time-temperature cycle for such a process is shown in Fig. 5.8 and the treatment is completed in 50 to 60 hours.

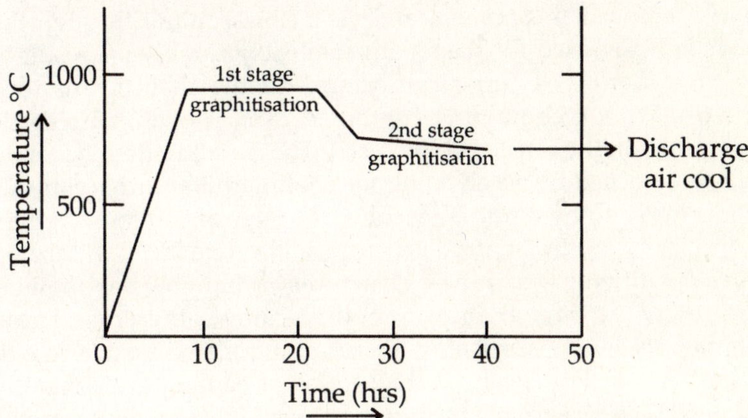

Fig. 5.8: Typical Time-Temperature cycle of a continuous white heart process[22]

5.5.2 Pearlitic Malleable Iron

As defined earlier, pearlitic malleable irons are those having a microstructure containing combined carbon in the matrix structure. Although these irons are designated as pearlitic, they may have pearlite, pearlite and ferrite, tempered martensite or spheroidal type of structure as the matrix. Such irons have superior strength and hardness than ferritic malleable irons because of the hardening effect of the carbide particles dispersed in the ferrite.

There are many variations in the procedures for the production of pearlitic malleable irons. Among these are:

1. Production by increasing the rate of cooling through and below the eutectoid range in order to avoid second stage graphitization (SSG).
2. Production by addition of alloying elements such as manganese, molybdenum or chromium to assist in retarding the second stage graphitization.
3. Production by cooling rapidly to avoid second stage graphitization followed by reheating to a temperature above the eutectoid zone, liquid quenching and then tempering.
4. Production by heat treatment of a completely graphitized ferritic malleable iron.

In the procedure (1), continuous and rapid cooling at various rates through the eutectoid transformation zone are substituted for the isothermal treatment and very slow cooling through the above zone as used for the ferritic malleable irons. As a result of this treatment, SSG does not occur and the resulting matrix structure is one containing combined carbon or is martensitic depending on the rate of cooling used. The desired rates of cooling may be obtained by accelerating the cooling in the furnace, by air quenching, and by liquid quenching. At rates of cooling less than the critical rate, the matrix structure will be pearlite of varying degree of fineness, or mixed structures containing pearlite and bainite etc. At higher rates of cooling above the critical rate obtained by liquid quenching, the resulting matrix structure will be martensite. However, the high rates of cooling are generally followed by tempering in the range of 230-700°C to relieve stresses and to obtain tempered martensite of the desired hardness. Further, if the final heating is close to 700°C and the heating is prolonged, a spheroidized structure consisting of spherical particles of carbide in a matrix of ferrite is obtained. The tempered martensite structures result in irons of maximum strength, hardness and wear resistance but low ductility. The spheroidized irons have superior ductility and better machinability than the lamellar pearlitic irons.

In method (2), additions of a carbide stabilizing element are made to aid in suppressing second stage graphitization. For example, addition of manganese between 0.5 to 0.9 per cent is made for this purpose. The presence of such elements serves to prevent graphitization during the spheroiding treatment some times employed as a part of procedure (1).

Procedure (3) is used to convert a pearlitic matrix to a tempered martensitic structure by heating to above the critical range, austenitizing, quenching to form martensite and tempering to get the desired hardness.

In the procedure (4), the fully graphitized ferritic castings are reheated to a temperature in the austenite range, held to dissolve sufficient temper carbon to provide the matrix structure and cooled at a appropriate rate to produce a desired structure and hardness. This procedure is employed in a plant normally making ferritic malleable irons to produce a limited amount of pearlitic irons.

It is thus obvious from above procedures that pearlitic malleable irons are essentially blackheart malleable irons to which a modified heat treatment cycle is applied to produce a structure having temper carbon in the matrix of pearlite or its other variations.

5.5.3 Heat Treatment Furnaces

Both batch type and continuous furnaces are used for annealing white iron castings to obtain malleable irons. Three types of batch furnaces are commonly used viz. pit type, elevator type and bell type. Continuous furnaces are employed for large scale production for example, for automobile castings.

The gaseous annealing processes reduce the total annealing time as these processes dispense with the cans and packing material. For malleabilizing white heart irons, controlled additions of air and steam is made to a sealed furnace to establish a suitable atmospheric condition. CO, CO_2, steam and hydrogen are the active constituents of the atmosphere used for white heart annealing. The inert and static atmosphere is used for black heart irons to ensure that no decarburization takes place. This is obtained by allowing the small amount of air locked inside the furnace to react with the carbon of the castings. The resulting atmosphere containing nitrogen, CO and CO_2 has the requisite characteristics. The same atmosphere is also suitable for pearlitic malleable irons. In the case of continuous furnaces for both the black heart ferritic and pearlitic malleable irons where the furnaces can not be completely sealed, a small amount of externally generated atmosphere may be necessary to combat inward air leakage. Use of nitrogen as inert atmosphere is also made in continuous annealing furnaces.

5.6 ENGINEERING PROPERTIES OF MALLEABLE IRONS

Mechanical Properties: The range of mechanical properties for both the ferritic and pearlitic malleable irons are given in the following table.

White heart ferritic malleable irons are relatively stronger and harder than black heart type. The pearlitic malleable irons are much stronger and harder than ferritic malleable irons with corresponding lower ductility. The greatest engineering value of malleable irons lies in the combination of their mechanical properties, service life, cost and suitability to many fabricating and processing operations. Among these advantages are :

Machinability: Malleable irons are among the most readily machinable of ferrous alloys. Moreover, because of the heat treatments done to all malleable iron castings, a high degree of uniformity of machinability is obtained during fabrication of these castings.

TABLE 5.2: MECHANICAL PROPERTIES OF FERRITIC AND PEARLITIC MALLEABLE IRONS

Tensile strength	–	50,000 to 100,000 or more psi (345 to 690 N/mm^2)
Yield strength	–	35,000 to 80,000 or more psi (241 to 552 N/mm^2)
Compression strength	–	greater than tensile strength
Elongation	–	20 to 2%
BHN	–	110 to 270
Modulus of elasticity intension	–	25×10^6 psi (17×10^4 N/mm^2)
Shear strength	–	0.80 of tensile strength
Endurance Ratio (Endurance Limit/Tensile Strength)	–	0.40-0.575

Ductility or Toughness: There are many processing operations such as coining, punching, press fitting, straightening etc. which require good ductility as provided by many grades of malleable irons. Similarly, there are also many applications where the castings are required to be deformed rather than fractured when over stressed. Malleable irons provide satisfactory performance in the above respect.

Wear Resistance: Many grades of malleable irons, particularly the pearlitic irons provide outstanding resistance in applications demanding the same. The ferritic grades however, do not have such inherent wear resistance but can be hardened by standard heat treatment to provide good wear resistance. The pearlitic irons respond readily to surface and localized hardening treatments for improved wear resistance.

Corrosion Resistance and Surface Coatings: Malleable irons also have excellent corrosion resistance and the latter may be greatly increased by providing surface coatings of zinc, aluminium and lead. For example, hot-dip galvanizing may be applied to clean malleable castings to provide good corrosion resistance to exposure in great variety of conditions or applications.

Magnetic Properties: The magnetic properties of all types of malleable irons are better than those of gray irons and are functions of their compositions. Upto field strength of 9000 or 10,000 gausses, malleable iron has properties superior to those of soft steels.

5.7 MALLEABLE IRON FOUNDRY PRACTICE

The first step in the manufacture of malleable iron castings of any type is production of white iron castings of suitable compositions. The manufacture of white iron castings involve the same foundry processes as used for other types of castings. Melting and pouring operations, moulding and core making, gating and risering, cleaning etc. are adopted to suit the foundry properties of the malleable irons (white cast irons) as discussed earlier.

5.7.1 Melting and Pouring

The melting is the first operation which converts the raw materials of the charge into a molten metal of proper temperature for pouring and of the desired chemical composition. The melting is accomplished by batch cold melting or by duplexing. The cold melting is done in air or rotary furnaces, direct arc furnaces, core less induction furnaces or cupola furnaces. In duplexing, the iron is melted in a cupola, core less induction furnace, or direct arc furnace and the molten metal is transferred to a air or rotary furnace, direct arc furnace or channel type induction furnace for refining and temperature control. Normally, duplex melting operations are carried out for the purpose of continuous melting. The details of these melting furnaces used either for batch melting or continuous melting have been given in Chapter 2.

The charge materials consist of mixtures of foundry malleable iron returns, steel scrap, ferroalloys and carbon (except, in case of cupola melting) carefully selected and added in suitable proportions to produce metals of desired compositions. The composition of charge constituents for a typical air furnace or rotary furnace melting operation can be:

Pig iron (malleable grade)	-	25-35%
Malleable foundry returns	-	45-55%
Malleable scrap	-	5-20%
Steel scrap	-	0-10%

Minor corrections in composition and pouring temperature are made in the second stage of duplex melting, but most of the process control is done in the primary melting furnace.

The pouring temperature for making a white iron casting varies depending upon section thickness of casting and composition of the iron in the range from 1425 to 1540° C which is substantially higher than those used for gray iron castings. The iron is taken from the melting furnace in overhead or buggy ladles and then transferred to pouring ladles at a location near the pouring station and poured into the moulds assembled there.

5.7.2 Moulding and Core Making

The technology of moulding and core making used in malleable iron foundry in general is similar to that used for gray iron castings for similar sizes and quantity of castings. However, since the white iron castings are susceptible to hot cracking, internal cores may be required to be especially collapsible. This may be achieved with core sands containing only organic binders and a minimum amount of core oil. Moulds are produced in green sand, silicate bonded CO_2 sand or resin bonded shell mould sands on equipment ranging from highly mechanized or automated machines to that required for floor or hand moulding methods, depending on the size and the number of the castings to be produced. Sands used for making moulds and cores are required to be more heat resistant because of higher pouring temperatures used for malleable irons.

Synthetic moulding sands are therefore generally used for this reason although some natural sands are employed.

Most malleable iron castings are light in weight generally less than 25 kg, although some casting may be quite heavy. The section thickness of light castings are correspondingly thin, generally less than 51 mm with a majority in the range of 4.8 mm to 38 mm.

5.7.3 Gating and Risering

The gates and sprues employed are usually large in size because of relatively high M.P. of the metal and its relatively more rapid solidification than those of higher carbon irons. The feeding problems of white iron castings have been already discussed and the various measures regarding appropriate size and position of the riser and the feeding aids like chills etc. are adopted.

5.7.4 Cleaning and Finishing

After the casting has solidified and cooled, the excess metal in the form of sprues, gates, feeders etc. are easily removed from the castings by impact i.e., by an operation called 'spruing' performed manually with a hammer. The foundry returns are then sent for melting and the castings are subjected to suitable heat treatment cycles. After the annealing, castings are cleaned and finished by grinding, tumbling, shot or grit blasting etc. The castings are then sent for painting, plating or any other finishing operations as may be required.

Spheroidal Graphite Cast Irons and Foundry Practice

6.1 INTRODUCTION

Spheroidal graphite cast iron is a revolutionary engineering material which combines the process advantages of gray cast iron (low melting point, good fluidity and castability) and product advantages of steel (high strength, toughness, ductility, hot workability and hardenability). It is variously reported in literature as ductile iron, nodular iron, spherulitic iron or spheriodal iron, but the ductile iron and the nodular iron are the most widely used terms. The term spheroidal graphite iron arises from the spherical shape of the graphite formed in the as-cast condition, a form which causes least interruption to the continuity of the metallic matrix and hence, has minimum detrimental effect on the matrix strength.

Spheriodal graphite (S.G.) irons are produced commercially by treating molten iron of appropriate composition with magnesium or cerium metal or complex alloys and materials containing these elements. The discovery of this new engineering material to the foundry industry was first announced in the year 1948 by the investigators[23,24] working independently in the United States and Great Britain, the International Nickel Company (INCO) and the British Cast Iron Research Association (BCIRA), respectively. Since its inception, S.G. irons have found numerous applications and are being produced in millions of tons all over the world.

Of the several cast ferrous metals, gray cast irons are the most popular because of their relative cheapness, favourable foundry characteristics and certain good engineering properties. However, their chief draw back has been their poor mechanical properties.

Although considerable research has been devoted and several measures have been taken to improve the strength of gray cast irons such as lowering of total carbon, inoculation and alloying and substantial success has been obtained in this respect. However, none of these improved higher strength gray irons have any significant ductility. Subsequently, the development of different types of malleable irons lead to enhanced mechanical properties with respect to strength and ductility. But a serious drawback of all the grades of malleable iron is the section thickness limitation besides the prolonged annealing cycle necessary. The S.G. cast iron in the as-cast condition, has strength much higher (40-45 tons/ in^2) than conventional gray iron (10-12 tons/in^2) and approaches that of cast-steel. The increased strength of S.G. irons is also accompanied by increase in toughness and ductility. The S.G. iron possesses the favourble fluidity and low melting point advantages of gray cast iron and does not suffer from section thickness limitation, as in the case of malleable irons. The mechanical properties of S.G. iron are almost similar to the mechanical properties of cast steel and it has an advantage over cast steel in that it possesses process advantages of gray cast iron due to its high carbon and silicon contents. The high fluidity of this material enables intricate and complex shapes to be readily cast. Its mechanical properties are distinctly superior to those of malleable irons. The superiority of S.G. irons over other ferrous cast alloys thus can best be expressed in the following worlds of Mr. W.W. Braidwood[25] : **"No steel has a freezing point temperature so low as 1150° C, no gray cast iron with such freezing point could ever exhibit an elongation of 20 per cent, and no malleable cast iron with such elongation could be cast in sections ranging from 1/8 to 40 inch or more, or could be cast with graphite in the as-cast condition, or could contain more than 3.5% C with over 2% Si. All these attributes are combined in S.G. iron".**

The production of S.G. cast iron throughout the world is increasing at a fast rate. This testifies its wide acceptance by the engineering industry. In advanced countries, the production of malleable castings is remaining static or declining whereas S.G. iron production is growing at the annual rate of 10 to 15% [26]. S.G. iron is not only replacing castings of other members of ferrous alloys such as malleable irons, gray iron and steel but also steel forgings and fabrications in many applications. Ductile iron has thus become a most popular engineering material with a worldwide market exceeding 16 million tons in 2004[26].

6.2 MANUFACTURE OF S.G. IRONS

As mentioned earlier, there are two basic processes of treating molten iron of suitable composition to get spheroidal graphite in the as-cast structure and which are also in use for production of S.G. cast irons i.e. INCO Process and BCIRA Process.

INCO Process: This process was developed by the Research Laboratory of the International Nickel Company, USA in which iron of a very wide composition range (including both the hypo- and hypereutectic compositions) is treated in the molten condition by addition of small amount of Mg or Mg along with other elements present in complex alloys.

BCIRA Process: This process was developed by British cast Iron Research Association of U.K. in which a small amount of Ce (0.02 to 0.2%) is added to the molten iron of higher carbon content (hyper eutectic compositions). The addition of cerium is made in the form of Misch metall, a mixture of rare earth compounds containing 40% of Ce. Besides Ce, this also contains the rare-earth metals like lanthanum, yttrium, samarium, neodymium and gadolinium.

Of the above two processes, the INCO Process of treating with magnesium has proved to be the most efficient and economic addition for industrial production and therefore most universally used. This process is also applicable to a wider range of composition of base iron. As such, this method of production of S.G. iron will be described in detail.

There are three basic steps involved in the production of S.G. cast irons:

1. Production of molten base iron of suitable composition
2. Treatment of the above iron with magnesium (popularly known as Mg treatment)
3. Post inoculation of the magnesium treated metal before pouring into the mould.

6.2.1 Production of Molten Base Iron

Molten iron of suitable composition and pouring temperature is first produced using different types of melting furnaces and post metal treating devices for desulfurization which will be discussed in detail under the subsequent section of melting practice.

6.2.1.1 Composition of Base Iron

The molten iron should have sulfur content as low as possible as sulfur will not only consume uselessly costly treating agent, but will also produce troublesome dross like MgS likely to be trapped as inclusions in the casting. Further, since good ductility is the characteristics of S.G. iron, the phosphorus content of the base iron should be also low as it forms brittle eutectic constituent, steadite which will lower the ductility and toughness of the cast product. In any case, it should not exceed 0.05%, if good low temperature impact properties are required.

The following range of chemical composition of the base iron suitable for magnesium treatment has been recommended :

Total carbon	:	3.0 to 4.20%, preferably 3.4 to 3.8%
Silicon	:	1.8 to 2.8%
Manganese	:	0.15 to 0.90
Phosphorus	:	0.05% maximum
Sulfur	:	0.03% maximum

The residual magnesium content after the treatment of the above metal for the effective spheroidization should be in the range of 0.02 to 0.08%. Besides Mg, other active elements like Ca or Ce may be also present and the residual contents of the same are recommended as Ce in the range of 0.02 to 0.03% and Ca in the range of 0.01 to 0.02%.

Besides the above desirable chemical composition, presence of certain elements even in trace amounts should be avoided because of their deleterious effect on the development of the spheroidal graphite structure. The presence of Pb, Ti, Al, Sb and Zr promotes formation of flake graphite. Similarly, As, B, Mn, Cr, Sn, Vd and even phosphorus are known to promote the formation of pearlite and/or iron carbide. Therefore, close control of composition over these elements is necessary. The following are the preferred maximum limits for the different undesirable trace elements[27]:

Pb	–	0.002%
Ti	–	0.03%
Sb	–	0.004%
Bi	–	0.002%
Zr	–	0.1%
Al	–	0.15%

6.2.1.2 Melting Practice

Selection of Raw Materials: In order to get control over tramp-element content, S.G. iron is prepared from melts using only selected steel scrap, special grades of pig iron (some foundries do not use at all or use only little pig iron) and foundry ductile return scrap. The purchased cast iron scrap is not used because the phosphorus content of such scrap is generally too high and other elements detrimental to production of S.G. iron are usually present in objectionable quantities. Most steel scrap available is higher in manganese content than is desirable for best mechanical properties of the as-cast metal, especially in light sections. Therefore, careful selection of steel scrap is also desirable.

Melting Furnaces: Various kinds of melting facilities are employed for producing base iron of desired composition. Acid cupola melting is the most common method used. About 75% of S.G. iron manufactures employ the acid cupola as the melting furnace since it is the most common available melting facility in many foundries which caters to the need of both gray iron and S.G. iron production. Acid cupola melting is also much less costly than basic cupola melting. However, its use necessitates close control over the charge materials like pig iron, scrap and coke. The sulfur content of the acid cupola metal is also high (0.06 to 0.12% S) and therefore needs external desulphurization in ladle using one of the different post metal treatment processes available and the basic materials such as soda ash, calcium carbide or quick lime to obtain sulfur content as low as 0.02% by above methods.

Basic cupola melting is preferred when new facilities are installed. Some 70 to 80% of the tonnage of S.G. iron produced is melted in basic cupolas which are capable of reducing sulfur content of the metal to as low value as 0.025 to 0.035%. However, such low content of sulfur is obtained at the expense of higher operating costs, higher silicon losses, less effective temperature and composition control and a greater carbon pick-up during melting. The use of water cooling and preheated blast therefore is adopted in basic cupola melting for better performance.

The current trend as well as the future trend is to use electric melting like coreless induction melting furnace, particularly the induction furnaces operating on mains frequency. Electric melting provides the best control over the compostion and temperature so that quality S.G. iron can be produced.

Besides the above primary melting furnaces, duplex melting practice using one of the systems like acid cupola + coreless or core type induction furnace, cupola + rotary furnace, direct arc furnace + core type induction furnace or coreless induction furnace + core type induction furnace, is also in use for producing base iron of desirable composition and temperature. The details of all above melting devices are described in the Chapter 2. Attempt is made to produce iron at higher temperatures in the range of 1400 to 1500° C suitable for treatment of this molten metal with spheroidizing agents.

6.2.2 Magnesium Treatment

The second step of the treatment of the molten base iron of suitable composition with magnesium or its other alloys is also known as SPHEROIDAZATION or NODULISING. The addition of pure magnesium in the molten iron involves technical difficulties due to (i) its high chemical activity; (ii) its low boiling point (1107° C); and (iii) its low specific gravity. Magnesium reacts with molten iron violently. It is vapourized and burns vigorously in air at the treatment temperatures which are usually 1400 to 1500° C. The vapourization of magnesium also produces a degassing effect removing the gasses dissolved in the metal. Due to its low specific gravity, it is difficult to plung it into the melt. Because of these reasons, special precautions are to be taken or special devices are to be adopted. To take care of the some of the above problems, magnesium is usually added in form of carrier alloys or master alloys which reduce the volatility of magnesium and also increase the bulk density. As such, besides pure magnesium, different types of alloys and materials containing magnesium are added for the treatment of the molten iron using a variety of special devices and processes.

6.2.2.1 Magnesium Treatment Agents

The following are different types of treating agents employed for nodulization[28-30]:

1. **Metallic Magnesium:** Pure magnesium is used in the form of powder, chippings, granules, ingots, rods, wires and compacts like briquettes.

2. **Carrier or Master Alloys:** Magnesium is added in the form of different alloys which may be divided into two groups depending on the specific gravity:
   (*i*) High specific gravity alloys like magnesium-nickel or copper alloys. Examples are Ni-20% Mg, Cu-15% Mg and lower cost alloys of Mg-Ni-Si containing 15% Mg, 50% Ni and 35% Si.
   (*ii*) Low specific gravity alloys like magnesium-ferrosilicon alloys containing 55% silicon, 5 to 35% Mg and small amounts of Ca, Ce and rare earths. In this category, there are also two groups, one group containing high amount of magnesium and the other group containing lower amount of magnesium (3 to 15% Mg).

3. **Reactive Slags or Salts:** Magnesium is also added in the form of reactive slags or salts of magnesium. Examples are-
   (*i*) Reactive slag consisting of Ca-Si together with chlorides or fluoride salts of Ca., Mg, Ce or rare earths.
   (*ii*) Mixture of salts of $MgCl_2$ and $CaCl_2$.

6.2.2.2 Magnesium Treatment Processes

A variety of magnesium treatment processes and devices have been developed and/or in use depending upon the type of the treatment agent used, number of S.G. iron castings required, and economic and other considerations. In general, what is desired that the method used should be simple, safe, reliable and economic besides giving good recovery of magnesium.

The various treatment processes available can be classified and discussed under the following main headings :

1. Processes for Metallic Magnesium
   (*i*) Pressure Ladle Process
   (*ii*) Pressure Chamber Process

(*iii*) Converter Process
(*iv*) Magnesium Wire Process
(*v*) Magnesium Impregnated Coke Process
(*vi*) Injection Process
(*vii*) Sprinkling Process

2. Processes for Magnesium Master Alloys with 5-35% Mg (Low Specific Gravity Alloys)

(*i*) Plunging Method
(*ii*) Rotating or Shaking Ladle Process
(*iii*) Injection Process
(*iv*) Sprinkling Process
(*v*) Mechanical Mixing Divices
(*vi*) Swedish Process (Ceramic Agitating Tube)
(*vii*) German Agitator

3. Processes for Magnesium Master Alloys with 3-15% Mg (Denser Alloys than type 2)

(*i*) Open Ladle or Pour Over Process
(*ii*) Sandwich Process
(*iii*) Lance Injection Process
(*iv*) Slag Sealed Process
(*v*) Flow-Through Vessel Processes
  (*a*) Flotret Process
  (*b*) Imconod Process
(*vi*) In Mould Process

4. Processes for Magnesium Master Alloys of High Specific Gravities

(*i*) Thrown in Ladle Process
(*ii*) Pour Over Method
(*iii*) Plunging Method

5. Processes for Reactive Slags or Salts of Magnesium and Calcium

(*i*) Reactive Slag Process
(*ii*) Slag Electrolysis Process

Magnesium Treatment Processes for Metallic Magnesium: It is difficult to add an element to a melt which is already above its boiling point (the vapourization point). Owing to its high volatility and oxidation-proneness, the addition of such element will be accompanied by substantial losses. For example, Mg has a much lower boiling point than the temperature at which molten iron is treated. The latter is of the order of 1400 to 1500° C and at such a temperature pure magnesium will give high vapour pressure of 6 to 10 atmosphere. Hence, inorder to retain its minimum residual content in the molten iron (necessary for spheroidization) and thus raise the recovery, magnesium is added under an over pressure (which raises the boiling point of the magnesium). For example, the volatilization of magnesium ceases at about 3 atmospheric pressure and therefore the magnesium treatment is carried out in pressure vessel devices at 2 to 4 atmospheric pressures.

In the Pressure Ladle (Autoclave) Process (Fig. 6.1), Mg is introduced into the pressure vessel separately and after closing the vessel, gas is admitted under such high pressure that the boiling point of Mg is raised well above the melt temperature. While this pressure is maintained, additives are mixed intimately with the melt by powerful agitation. A modified version of the above process is the Pressure Chamber Process, in which no special ladle is employed. A normal ladle is placed inside a pressure chamber and magnesium is introduced with a plunger under pressure.

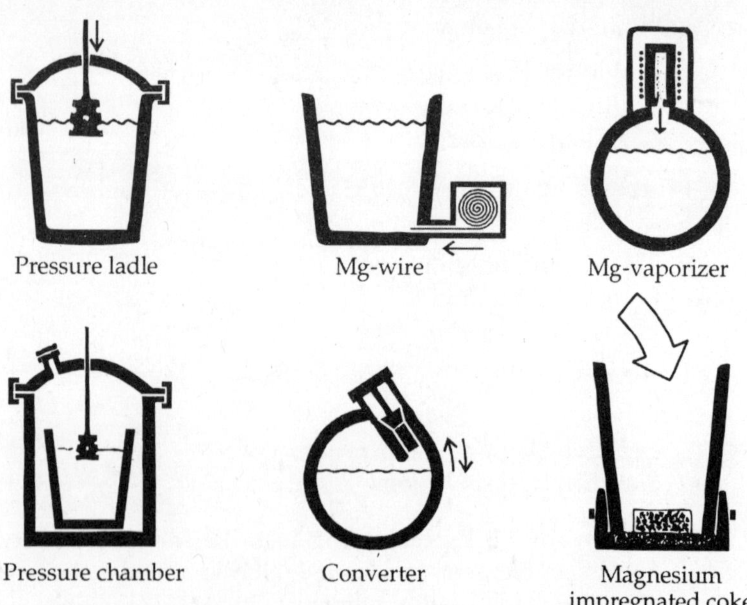

Fig. 6.1: Magnesium Treatment Processes for Introducing Metallic Magnesium

Another variant of the above processes uses Converters of different designs in which magnesium is vapourized under pressure and brought into intimate contact with the melt. In the Russian practice, inductively heated magnesium vapourizers are placed upon pressure ladles or converters so that dosed quantities of magnesium vapour are fed into the melt. In this way, large quantities of the molten iron from 50 to 100 tons or more can be treated.

An older process is the Magnesium Wire Method by which magnesium wire is fed into the melt through a ceramic gland close to the bottom of the ladle. The molten magnesium can be also introduced into the melt under pressure through a ceramic foot valve. One of the best established processes, uses a converter in which ingots of magnesium are introduced into the bottom of the liquid metal in a tiltable-vessel under atmospheric pressure. Other methods have been also designed for introducing magnesium powder or rods into the molten metal with atmospheric or pressurized vessels designed to exclude air and to prevent the ejection of the molten metal and fumes during the solution of the magnesium.

Magnesium particles have been made into different types of compacts with iron powder or swarf which reduce somewhat the violence of the reaction. Such materials are added in special vessels or by plunging into the ladle in a refractory bell. In another technique, popular in USA, Magnesium-Impregnated Coke containing 43% Mg is used to nodulize the graphite. Plunging such material into the molten iron results in a slow evolution of magnesium vapour from the pores of the coke into the iron. After the ladle treatment, the coke floats easily on the surface of the melt and helps removal of the slag and the reaction products during skimming. This process a quite economic, since the coke is much cheapter than the 'carrier metals' like nickel or silicon.

Injection Processes are also suited for introducing pure magnesium powder into the melt through a graphite tube using a carrier gas like nitrogen. Then, there is also a sprinkling method (Fig. 6.2) by which magnesium powder is sprinkled onto the surface of the melt. By admitting a inert gas at the same time through a porous plug brick, a strong movement is set up in the iron bath ensuring good mixing of the magnesium powder with the melt.

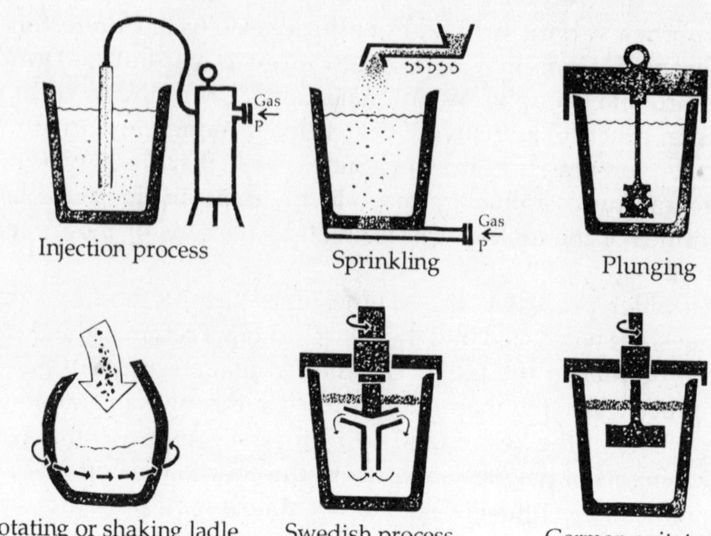

Fig. 6.2: Magnesium Treatment Processes for Low Specific Gravity Master Alloys Containing 5 to 35% Mg

Magnesium Treatment Processes for Low Specific Gravity Master Alloys containing 5 to 35% Mg: For economic reasons, the use of cheaper master alloys based on ferrosilicon has assumed a dominating position. These alloys consist of ferro-silicon containing magnesium and usually calcium and cerium as well. One very popular process used in Europe is the Plunging Method which makes use of a tall, narrow ladle (having height to diameter ratio to 2:1) with a heavy cast iron lid in which a plunger of refractory material or graphite is suspended along with the master alloy. Alternatively, the master alloy containing 35% Mg is placed into a perforated graphite or refractory bell shaped container or basket fastened to the plunging rod. The alloy is then plunged into the melt. A strong reaction occurs, bringing an effective purificatiion of the melt from inclusions besides inducing the formation of the spheroidal graphite. Very consistent and high recovery is obtained.

When large quantities of ductile iron are to be produced, Shaking or Rotating Ladle Processes (Fig. 6.2) are considered to be superior to the Plunging Method. The bath movement essential for good mixing of the melt is obtained in these processes by making the ladle revolve about its axis or else by using a shaking ladle that set up a sort of surf action in the bath with waves breaking over each other.

In the shaking or rotating ladles it is possible to use the master alloy of high specific weight as well as the lighter MgSi alloys with 5 to 15% Mg. Injection as well as sprinkling processes, as described above for pure magnesium are also suitable for treatment with such master alloys.

In order to obtain a fast and intimate mixing, Mechanical Mixing Devices are also employed. These include a Swedish Process, which uses a ceramic agitating tube to set up strong turbulence in the melt, and a German Agitator, which also ensures effective movement in the bath.

Magnesium Treatment Processes for Low Specific Gravity Master Alloys containing 3 to 15% Mg: For such master alloys, the economic Pour-Over Method (Fig. 6.3) has been accepted in various quarters. Here, the master alloy, e.g. a MgSiFe master alloy with 5 to 15% Mg is heaped one side on the bottom of the treatment ladle, covered over with clean sheet iron, after which the iron is poured into the opposite side of the ladle so that it spreads slowly over the covered master alloy. As the ladle is filled, the magnesium reaction commences and proceeds mildly and takes 20 to 120 seconds for completion depending on the quantity used.

A Sandwich Process evolved in USA and also known as Ladle-Pocket Method consists of placing the master alloy into a recession in the bottom of ladle. The alloy is then covered by a steel plate, sheet iron or iron chips, ferrosilicon (as inoculant) or inert material such as sand before tapping. In this way, the reaction time between magnesium and the iron is delayed until the ladle is at least partially filled with the metal thus increasing the magnesium recovery comparable to Plunging Method. Most of the master alloys used are based on FeSi containing 3 to 10% Mg. The reaction varies from fairly violent (with 10% Mg) to quite (with 3% Mg) and thus the efficiency of Mg recovery increases as the magnesium content of the alloy is reduced.

Another European method based on the use of master alloys of low magnesium contest (5 to 10% Mg) uses the alloy in the powder form. In this method (Fig. 6.3), the alloy is fed into the hollow stream of the molten iron formed by a ceramic orifice of a nozzle box placed over the pouring ladle. Through this device, the master alloy trickles down into the middle of the stream and the reaction is completed at the end of the hollow jet.

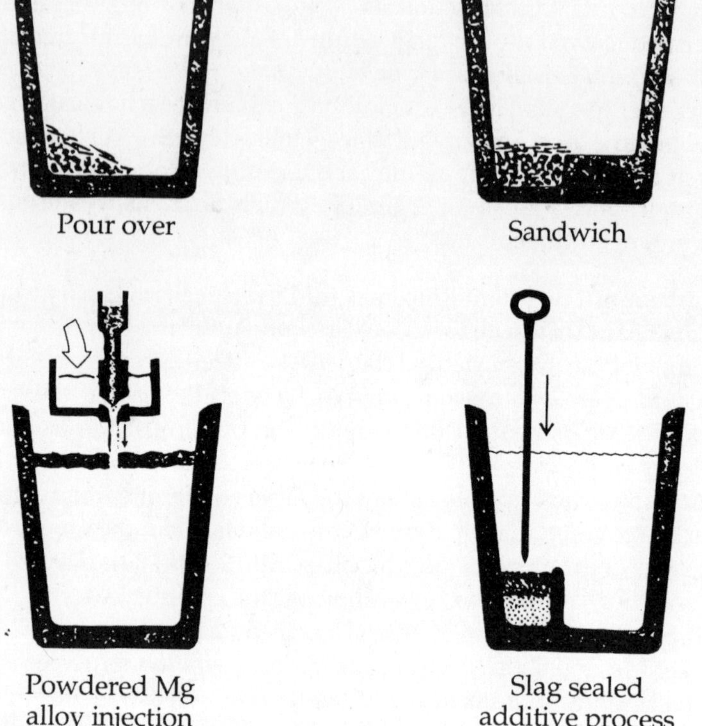

Fig. 6.3: Magnesium Treatment Processes for Low Specific Gravity Master Alloys Containing 3 to 15% Mg

In a process known as Slag-Sealed Process, a magnesium master alloy containing 5% Mg (and of grain size 0-1 mm) is placed in a recess in the bottom of a conventional ladle and is covered with a layer of fine powder of calcium carbide. As the metal from the furnace is tapped into the ladle, it forms with the calcium carbide a sticky slag over the top of the magnesium addition and prevents contact between the alloy and the metal. The ladle is filled to the normal height and after the tapping is finished, it is conveyed to the area for pouring the castings. At an appropriate stage, a steel rod is thrust down to the bottom of the ladle to break the slag crust formed and thereby allowing the metal to make contact with the master alloy and set off the reaction. Very little reaction violence occurs and good recoveries of magnesium are obtained. This process is in regular use by several German foundries.

Besides above processes, there are several other methods in use in which the molten iron is treated as it fills the ladle. The Flotret Process consists of placing the master alloy in a cavity in a closed vessel through which the molten metal is poured between the furnace and the ladle. This method can be used when pouring metal from one ladle to another ladle. Another design of such flow-through vessel is used in the process called as Imconod Process. The mater alloy can be also placed inside a mould (known as Inmould Process) while the metal is poured into the mould. The alloy is placed in a specially designed chamber or enlargement of the running system before closing the mould and alloy dissolves as the metal is cast. This method contains the reaction in the mould and avoids ejection of fume and flame.

Magnesium Treatment Processes for Heavy Master Alloys: Under this category, the examples of carrier alloys are Ni-Mg, Cu-Mg and Ni-Si-Mg alloys. Such heavy master alloys may either be placed on the bottom of the ladle (Pour Over Process) or Thrown into the melt (Thrown in Ladle Process) after which they sink to the bottom (Fig. 6.4). A mild reaction occurs and the dissolution of the master alloy is easier to control than pure magnesium. The Ni-Mg or Ni-Cu alloys are costlier than magnesium master alloys free of Ni or Cu. However, Ni-Mg master alloys have been in use since the beginning of S.G. iron production both in U.S.A. and U.K. besides other countries which also use them to a limited extent.

Magnesium Treatment Processes Using Reactive Slags or Salts: Treatment with Reactive Slags (a Japanese Process) consists of placing (Fig. 6.5) the slag on the surface of the melt and stirring into it mechanically during which the reaction with the molten metal occurs. The treatment agent consists of granular, calcium-silicon coated with a flux and contains 3% Mg along with the rare earths for neutralizing tramp elements. However, reactive slags consisting of a mixture of calcium-silicon with the fluorides or halides of the rare earths with or without magnesium are also found suitable for producing small castings in small numbers. When such slags are placed over the melt, the calcium reacts with the halides of the rare earths, forming calcium halides and releasing the rare earths. The latter diffuse into the iron melt and promote the formation of spheroidal graphite. Because this reaction proceeds underneath the slag layer, losses of rare earth metals are minimum. Further, fewer non-metallic inclusions of metal oxides are formed. Another advantage lies in the exothermic slag reaction which ensures that the temperature drop in the melt during the treatment is very slight.

In the Slag Electrolysis Process (Fig. 6.5), the active elements for spheroidal graphite formation are reduced into the melt from a reactive slag consisting mainly of magnesium and calcium chloride, besides small amounts of cerium chloride or fluoride, by the electrolysis carried out at temperatures of 1360 to 1370°C in a basic lined electric furnace. This process can be also operated continuously.

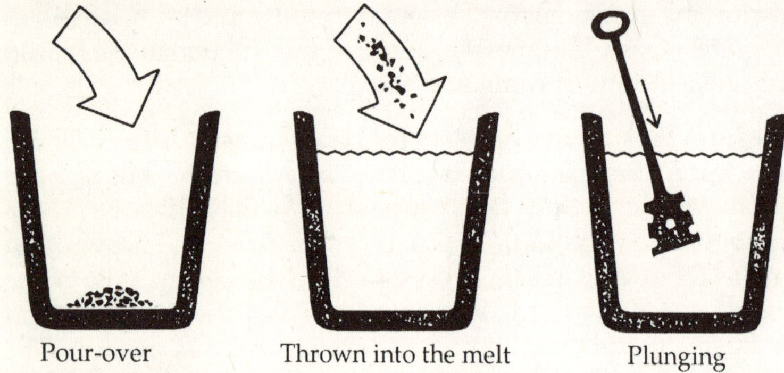

Fig. 6.4: Magnesium Treatment Processes for Heavy Master Alloys

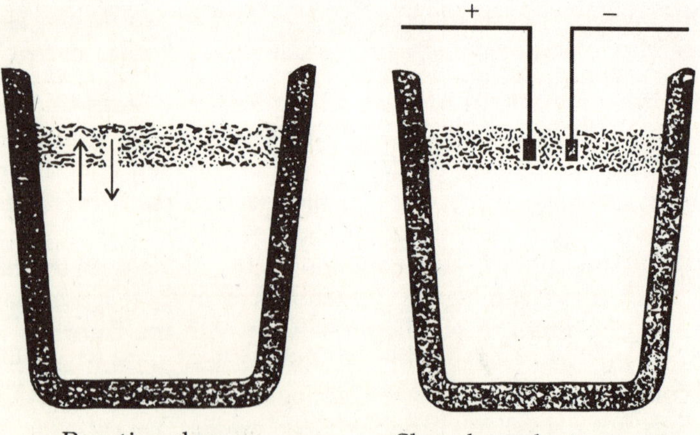

Fig. 6.5: Magnesium Treatment Processes using Reactive Slags or Salts

Magnesium Treatment Amount, Temperature, Time and Recovery: For the various processes as described above, the amounts of the master alloy to be added must be determined to ensure a residual magnesium content of 0.02 to 0.08% in the S.G. iron, making allowance for the initial sulfur content and the treatment temperature as well as the standing time before pouring. In practice, master alloys amounting to 0.8 to 2.5% of the melt weight are added. The treatment temperature and time also vary from 1400 to 1500°C (preferably 1450 to 1500° C) and 20 seconds to 2 minutes, respectively.

The recovery of magnesium depends upon a number of factors such as type of the master alloy and its magnesium content, the method of addition and equipment employed, the temperature of the iron, the sulfur content of the iron and other circumstantial factors like the depth of the liquid iron through which the magnesium vapour rises before entering the atmosphere, the time required to cover the carrier alloy and the depth to which it is covered etc. It varies from 25 to 50 percent depending on the above factors.

6.2.3 Inoculation (Also Called Post-Inoculation)

The introduction of magnesium into the base iron is followed by inoculation which refers to the practice of making an addition to the magnesium treated metal which will increase the number of spheroids formed during solidification. The purpose of inoculation is to provide a large number of sites from which graphite nodules can grow in order to prevent the formation of eutectic carbides and to produce a structure which contains an even distribution of small, well formed nodules. The iron must be poured as soon as possible after the inoculation so that the effects of both the magnesium and inoculant fade are minimized.

The most effective inoculants used are Fe-Si alloys. The other inoculants added are Ca-bearing Fe-Si, calcium-silicon alloy or various combinations of these. The common grades of Fe-Si alloys used contain 75 or 85% silicon and approximately 0.5 to 1.5% Si as Fe-Si is added into the melt.

The effective inoculation can be made by:

1. Reladling the metal after magnesium treatment and adding the inoculant as the metal is poured

2. Adding magnesium to the first half of the tap or pour and then adding inoculant to the last half.
3. Stirring the inoculant into the magnesium treated melt or
4. A combination of the last two methods
5. Sometimes inoculant is placed in the sprue base of the gating system of the mould and the metal is inoculated while being poured into the mould through it.

The silicon content of the inoculated iron increases by 0.30 to 0.70% and therefore the silicon content of the base iron is kept low so that silicon increase from addition of magnesium treating alloy and the inoculant adjust the final content to the desired value in the final composition of the S.G. iron.

6.3 SOLIDIFICATION OF S.G. IRON

Although the base chemistry of gray and ductile iron is essentially the same (with the exception of oxygen, sulfur and magnesium contents) these alloys solidify according to quite different modes. The gray iron of eutectic composition solidifies in more or less conventional manner with the combined or cooperative growth of austenite and graphite both in contact with the eutectic liquid and the solidification proceeds by the growth of eutectic cells of austenite and flake graphite over a temperature range. Further cooling of completely solidified alloy results in rejection of carbon from the solid austenite and precipitation of graphite on the preexisting graphite flakes. This process continues until eutectoid temperature range is attained cooling through which will result in variety of matrix structures ranging from all ferrite to all pearlite depending on rate of cooling and/or alloying elements present.

In contrast to above, ductile iron solidifies with completely divorced eutectic growth i.e. the graphite and austenite phases crystallize separately (they nucleate independently with respect to time and space) with the considerable under cooling of the melt[34]. It is now confirmed[35] that spheroidal graphite formation takes place by direct precipitation of carbon from the carbon saturated iron melt at suitable sites within the melt, provided by the inoculant addition and the graphite grows in direct contact with the melt at least in the initial stages of nodule formation. Thus, there can be two stages of nodule formation. In the first stage, after nucleation, as the growth of the nodules continues, the remaining iron, now lower in carbon forms a "halo or shell" around the nodule which shows an increasing tendency to solidify as the nodule size increases[36]. This halo layer produces the austenite shell and its thickness is determined by the rate of solidification (Fig. 6.6).

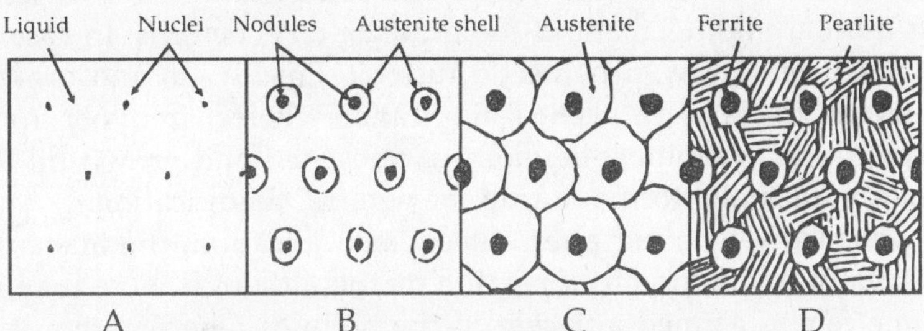

Fig. 6.6: Stages in the Formation of Austenite-Nodular Graphite Eutectic Cell (Courtesy of Portcullis Press, Redhill).

The second stage of solidification begins after the nucleation and solidification of the halo of austenite which considerably slows down the growth of the nodules of graphite. During this stage, the austenite shell grows slightly in contact with the liquid. In most cases, solidification is completed during this stage, but it is also possible that the existing nodules may grow a little further either as a result of carbon diffusion through austenite shell or mainly by transformation of austenite to ferrite during cooling and thereby leading to deposition of carbon on the nodule.

However, a larger number of nodule count i.e. the number graphite-austenite eutectic cells (graphite surrounded by austenite) per unit area formed in case of ductile iron than that of gray iron can be explained on the basis of the fact that since the graphite growth is brought to a stand still by the surrouding austenite shell, new graphite nuclei must appear continually to provide for the precipitation of the all the carbon present in the melt. This second stage of nodules formation also explains why the liquid metal is found to be present over a wider temperature range and to lower temperature for ductile iron solidification than for gray iron.

Treating of the iron melt with nodulizing elements like Mg, etc. suppresses the combined or cooperative growth of the iron and graphite (as obtained in gray iron) and solidification occurs in accordance with a divorced eutectic growth reaction in which the iron and graphite phases form independently[37]. This type of solidification in which only one phase i.e. austenite is in contact with the liquid after enveloping graphite nodule is known as Neoeutectic solidification. The growth of each eutectic cell takes place by the movement of carbon atoms from the liquid through the austenite shell to the nodule and solidification is completed on mutual impingement of the growing eutectic cells. In case of hypoeutectic irons, proeutectic austenite nucleation and growth precedes the above eutectic solidification whereas in hyper irons, proeutectic graphite spheroids are nucleated and grown till the halo of austenite forms during the eutectic solidification.

On further cooling after eutectic solidification, the austenite normally transforms to a pearlite matrix although there may be some ferrite formed adjacent to the nodules where carbon has left the austenite to deposit on the graphite. Fully ferritic matrix structures can be obtained in the as-cast condition by the use of high carbon and silicon contents and by avoidance of pearlite formers such as manganese, chromium and trace elements.

6.4 MECHANISM OF SPHEROIDAL GRAPHITE FORMATION

Gray cast iron contains comparatively large quantities of sulfur and oxygen whereas S.G. iron is thoroughly desulphurized, deoxidized and it contains free and uncombined magnesium which promotes formation of spheroidal graphite. This difference between the two irons shows up in increased undercooling of the eutectic melt during solidification leading to chilling tendency in thin and medium section thicknesses unless inoculation with FeSi follows magnesium treatment.

The following Fig. 6.7 illustrates the undercooling behaviour of both type of irons[38]. It shows the liquidus and solidus temperature of the inoculated and uninoculated iron melts at various degrees of saturation. The equilibrium temperature of eutectic solidification is plotted in this figure in order that the undercooling may be taken as the difference between the equilibrium temperature and the measured solidus temperature. It is now further confirmed[39] that high surface tension which is indicative of a high melt purity as well as supercooling during solidification are the main conditions which promote spheroidization of graphite.

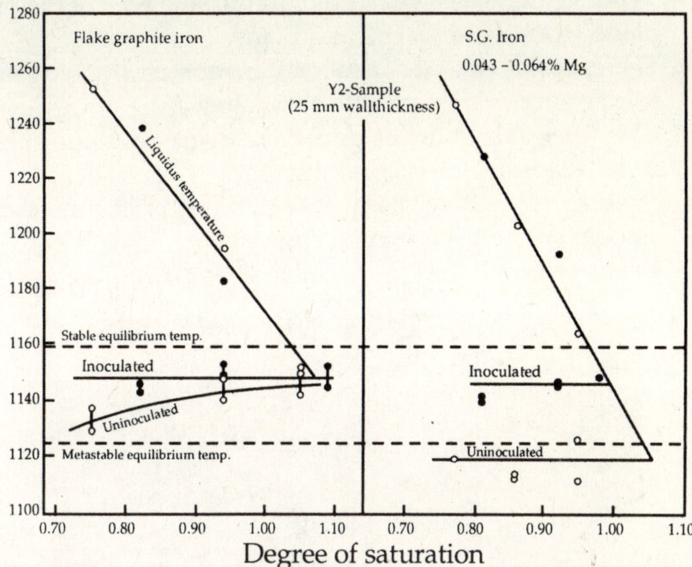

Fig. 6.7: Liquidus and Solidus Temperatures of Inoculated and Uninoculated Gray and S.G. Cast Iron Melts as a Function of Degree of Saturation

Fig. 6.8 shows the appearance and structure of a graphite spheroid as seen under the microscope in a sample of spheroidal graphite iron produced by magnesium treatment process. A more general view of graphite spheroids in a ferritic matrix is shown in Fig. 6.9. It is not yet clearly known that why magnesium or cerium additions to suitable molten base iron compositions can cause spheroidization of graphite, but a number of explanations have been suggested. Several authors have reviewed the theories put forward[34, 40–42]. Among the theories postulated to account for spheroid formation are the following :

1. Graphite nodules form as a result of an attempt of the melt to minimize its free energy by minimizing graphite-melt interfacial area.
2. Nodule formation depends on the absence of certain surface-active elements which alter the growth direction of graphite from the pole of the basal plane to the pole of the prism plane.
3. Nodule growth depends on surface adsorption of the nodulizing addition onto the graphite lattice which causes

a change in the growth direction from the pole of the prism plane to the pole of the basal plane.

4. The graphite growth direction depends on the type of the nuclei upon which growth is initiated.
5. Graphite nodules must grow within an austenite shell or from supersaturated austenite.
6. Nodules form as a consequence of non-equilibrium growth associated with the under cooling.
7. Graphite nodules form in gas bubbles within the melt.

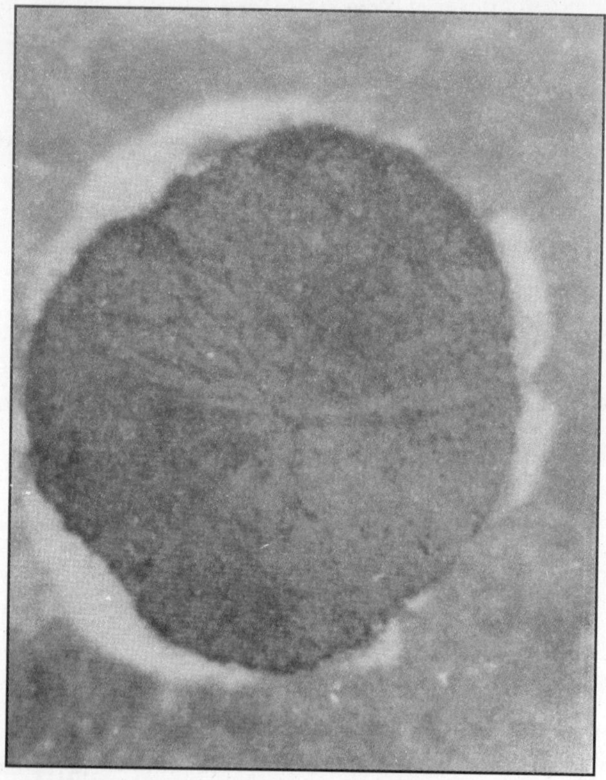

Fig. 6.8: Appearance and Structure of a Graphite Spheroid as seen under the Microscope (From J. H. Frencis, Applied Science in the Casting of Metals (ed. K. Strauss), Pergamon Press Oxford, 1970, p. 200).

Among the different theories postulated, those related to surface properties of the melt appear to be the most feasible. Many investigators have reported the detrimental effects of the elements

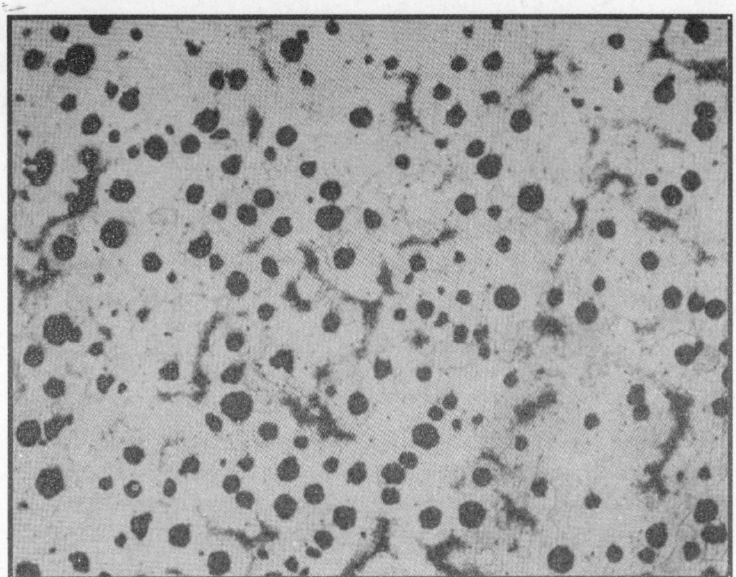

Fig. 6.9: A General View of Graphite Spheroids in a Ferritic Matrix (From J. H. Frencis, Applied Science in the Casting of Metals (ed. K. Strauss), Pergamon Press Oxford, 1970, p. 200)

in the melt (like O, S etc.) that lower the surface tension and the beneficial effects of eliminating surface-active elements or of adding elements that raise the surface tension. This suggests that in melts with a high surface tension, nodular graphite growth may either be a consequence of an attempt to minimize the surface area of the graphite and thus minimize the total free energy of the melt system, or that the nodular graphite results from the absence of certain elements that adsorb onto the graphite lattice and change the interfacial energy and the growth mode.

The former theory can be simply explained as the addition of Mg, Ce etc. to the iron melt removes oxygen and sulfur like impurities which will otherwise decrease the surface tension of the molten iron by segregation in the melt surface. Therefore, by their removal the interfacial surface tension between graphite particles and the melt increases which constraints the graphite to decrease its surface area per unit volume which is done by acquiring a spherical shape.

Regarding the second alternative i.e. the change in the interfacial energy and the growth mode, it can be explained with the help of the Fig. 6.10 schematically illustrating the mode of growth of the graphite[40]. When sulfur and other surface-active elements are present, they are preferentially adsorbed onto the normally high energy prism planes and reduce the prism plane interfacial energy with the melt to a value below that for the basal planes. The result is a change in growth direction to the pole of the planes with the lowest interfacial energy i.e. the prism planes. Propagation of the low energy planes into the melt produces a melt-graphite system with the lowest total free energy i.e. the formation of flake type graphite takes place.

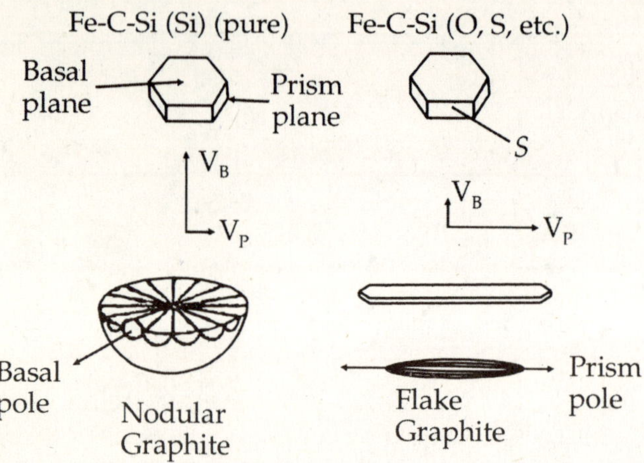

Fig. 6.10: Graphite Growth Morphologies for Spheroidal and Flake Graphite[40]

In the absence of surface-active elements, carbon atoms are preferentially added to the basal plane, perhaps on screw dislocations. The low energy basal plane propagates along its pole and produces the lowest free energy melt-graphite configuration. The function of nodulizing additions like Mg, Ce etc. is to scavenge the melt of free surface-active elements capable of preferentially adsorbing on the graphite prism plane. In the absence of surface-active elements, the basal plane has the lowest surface energy in contact with the melt and grows to produce spheroidal graphite.

The theory put forward in terms of nucleation of graphite spheroids by tiny bubbles of gas can be explained as follows[43]. The molten iron contains ample hydrogen to form very large numbers of microscopic bubbles which can form nuclei for the formation of graphite spheroids since they already have their interior lined with the carbon obtained from the reaction with added magnesium as:

$$\text{Mg vapour} + \text{CO gas} = \text{MgO solid} + \text{C solid}$$

The carbon can penetrate inside these bubbles and completely fill them. The graphite burns oxygen present in the melt to form CO gas required for the above reaction. The alkali earth metals employed successfully as nodulizers, all have the property of being able to absorb large quantities of hydrogen at room temperature and liberate it when the temperature is raised. When they are immersed in the molten iron, microscopic bubbles are evolved which form nuclei for the rapidly diffusing carbon which remains as spheroids after the iron solidifies.

A significant amount of research work has been done regarding the source of nucleation of the spheroidal graphite. In a recent investigation covering the nucleation of such graphite, Lalich and Hitchings[44] have confirmed the findings of other investigators by demonstrating the importance of non-metallic inclusions. For example, they have found that compounds of magnesium calcium sulfied acted as heterogeneous nuclei for graphite nodules in S.G. cast irons made from magnesium ferrosilicon treatment alloys (Fig. 6.11). They concluded from the evidence obtained in their research that the majority of the spheroids of graphite in S.G. irons is associated with nonmetallic inclusions and that graphite growth in some instances is related to the shape and distribution of the nonmetallic inclusions.

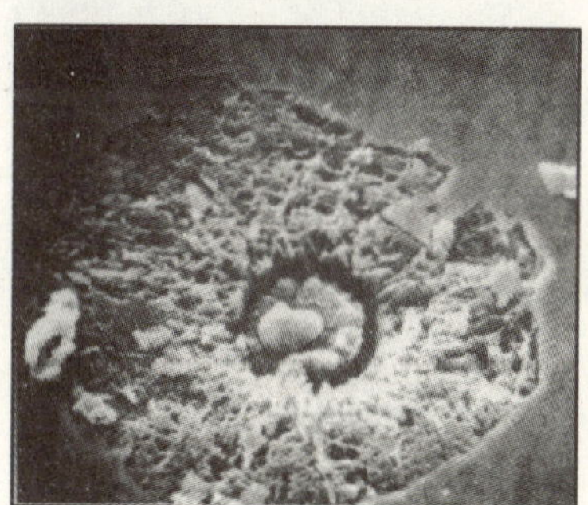

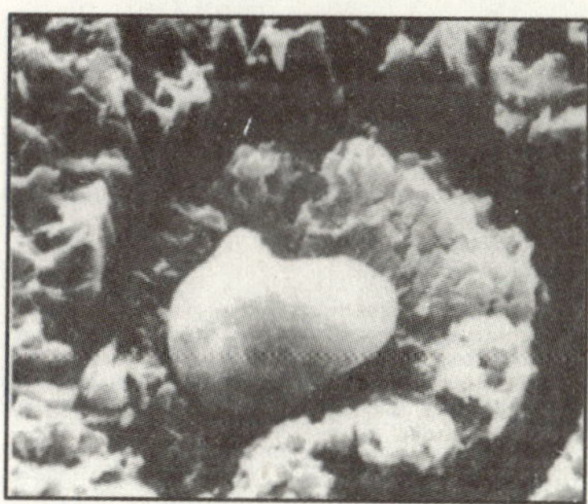

Fig. 6.11: Magnesium-Calcium Sulfide Nucleus in Graphite Nodules[44] (Plasma etch), (*a*) X 2500, (*b*) X 10,000

In general, the amount of nodulizer added must not exceed certain limits as recommended earlier since in many cases, this leads to cementite formation. However, a small residual content must also remain in the melt for optimum spheroidization. Under commercial conditions, the effect of all nodulizers fades with time due to burn-off these elements, evaporation losses and reaction with crucible lining and therefore metal should be poured quickly in the moulds after magnesium treatment and post inoculation.

6.5 STRUCTURE, PROPERTIES AND APPLICATIONS OF S.G. IRONS

6.5.1 Microstructure

As-cast matrix structure of unalloyed S.G. cast iron is generally pearlite or pearlite and ferrite. This matrix structure may be converted to all ferrite by annealing or to martensite and tempered martensite by heat treatment as indicated in Fig. 6.12a-c. The as-cast structure of the S.G. iron resembles that of a pearlitic malleable iron (Fig. 6.12a, a Bull's eye structure) with the graphite inclusion approaching a more nearly spheroidal shape than is ordinarily the case with malleable microstructures.

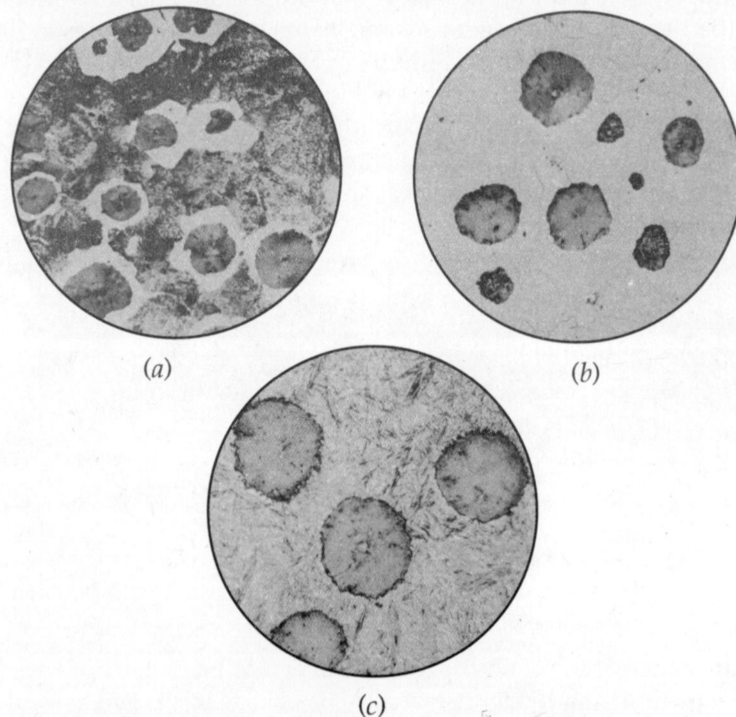

(*a*) (*b*) (*c*)

Fig. 6.12: Microstructures of S.G. Irons (*a*) Top-As-cast, 250X, (*b*) Middle-Annealed 250X, (*c*) Bottom-Quenched and Tempered, 340X. (From *The Cupola and its Operation*, AFS, Illinois, 1965, p. 319).

Besides the spherical shape of graphite, other shapes of graphite may also develop (Fig. 6.13) if the manufacturing process is not carried out properly. The graphite shape is dependent on pouring temperature, casting section size, amount of nodulizer added, post inoculation and the base analysis of iron. In general, the poorer graphite shapes are developed with low pouring temperature, heavy section sizes, insufficient magnesium addition, lack of inoculation and low carbon equivalent.

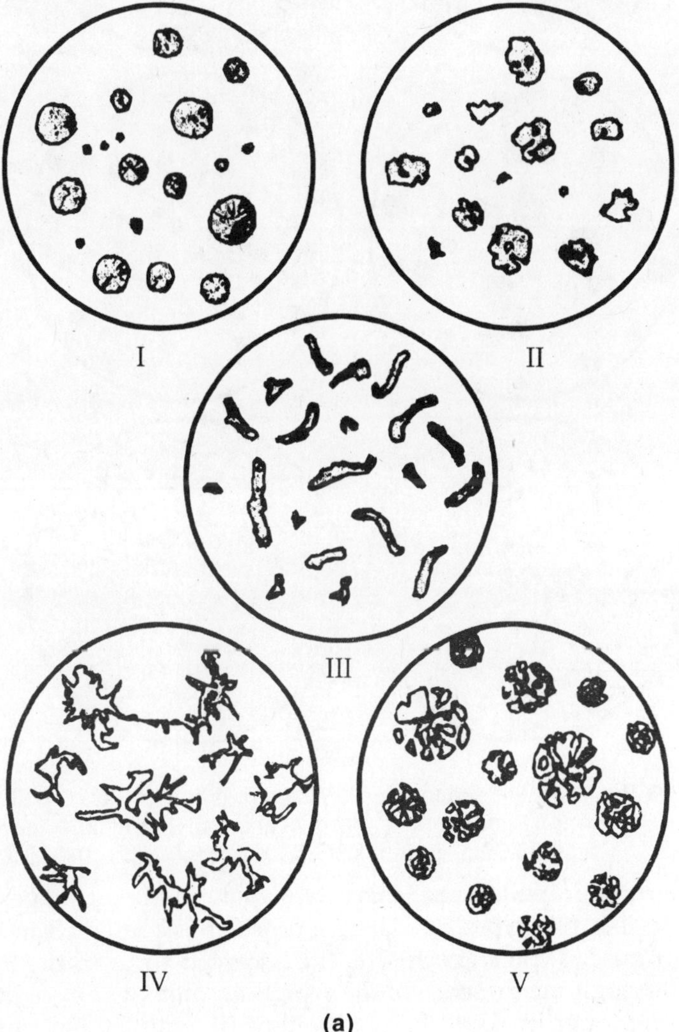

(a)

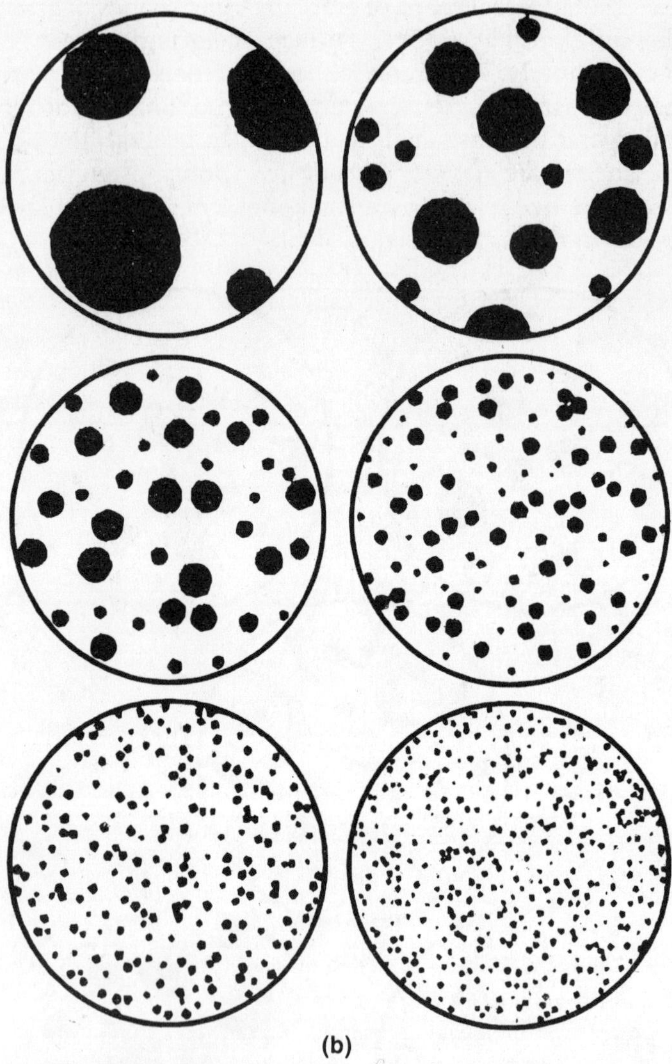

(b)

Fig. 6.13 (b): Different shapes and of sizes graphite in S.G. Cast Iron, X100 (From W. Heine, R. Loper and P. C. Rosenthal, Principles of Metal Casting, Tata McGraw Hill, New Delhi, 1976, p. 629)

Like flake graphite irons, charts classifying different shapes of graphite into five types have been proposed as presented in the above figure. Type I graphite is the accepted form in the S.G. iron, although the presence of the type II graphite will have little effect on properties. Upto 10% of the type III, with the remaining graphite as type I or II has been reported to have no noticeable effect on properties. Increased amount of type III graphite are not desirable. Types IV or V are most undesirable and significantly lower the mechanical properties of the S.G. irons. Besides the above five types of graphite, some six sizes of graphite spheroids have been also proposed (Fig. 6.13b).

In high-carbon equivalent S.G. irons, particularly with over 4.6% carbon equivalent, graphite flotation may occur during solidification and the formation of the exploded graphite, type V may occur. This problem is magnified by heavy section size of the casting. Such graphite flotation may occur, since the graphite formed early in the solidification process rapidly grows to a large size in the above type irons and thus becomes buoyant and floats to the cope surface. Such form of graphite leads to considerable deterioration in properties.

6.5.2 Engineering Properties

Mechanical Properties: The following table gives the range of the mechanical properties of the unalloyed S.G. irons:

TABLE 6.1: MECHANICAL PROPERTIES OF S.G. IRONS

Tensile Strength	–	60,000 to 150,000 psi(414 to 1034, N/mm^2)
Yield Strength	–	40,000 to 120,000 psi(380 to 838 N/mm^2)
Elongation	–	25-2%
Modulus of Elasticity in Tension	–	22,000,000 to 25,000,000 psi(1517,000 to 1724,000 N/mm^2)
BHN	–	130-340
Endurance Ratio (Ratio of Endurance Limit/Tensile Strength)	–	0.35-0.55
Ratio of Sheer Strength in Tension to Tensile Strength	–	0.90

Lower tensile and yield strengths with high ductilities are obtainable with ferritic matrix. The higher tensile and yield strengths and lower ductilities are obtained in pearlitic grades. Further, higher strength levels are attained by quenching and tempering.

The presence of graphite in the spheroidal condition results in a minimum interruption of the matrix of the S.G. irons as opposed to that of flake graphite irons, where the matrix continuity is reduced by the flattened graphite flakes (Fig. 6.14). Hence, ductilities ranging from 2 to 25% are obtained in S.G. irons as opposed to the near zero ductility of gray irons. In general, the mechanical properties of S.G. irons are similar to that of cast steels and distinctly superior to that of malleable irons.

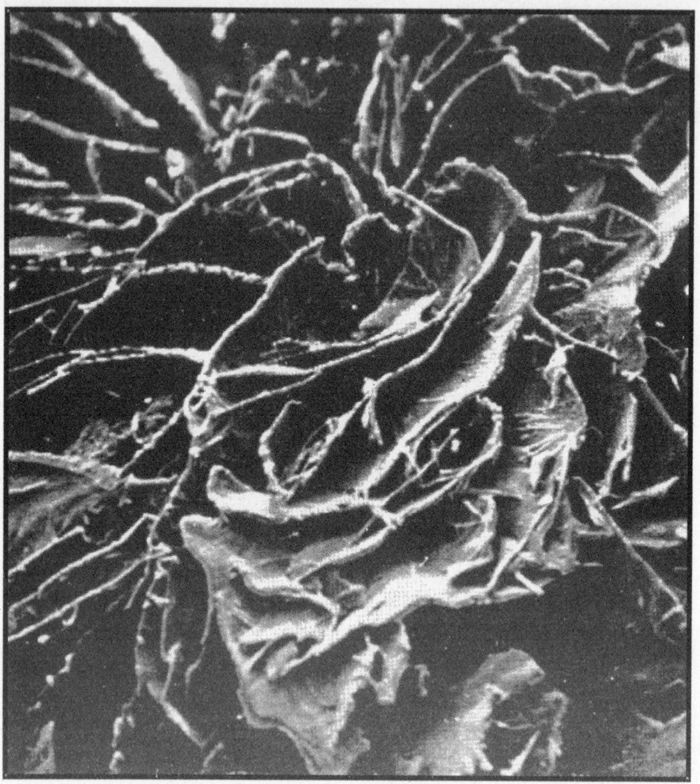

Fig. 6.14: Scanning Electron Microscopic View of Eutectic Graphite in Gray Iron, X400 (Courtesy of Portcullis Press, Redhill).

Machinability: The machinability of S.G. iron is superior to that of gray iron at equivalent hardness and better than that of steel at equivalent strength levels.

Damping Capacity: S.G. iron has significantly higher damping capacity compared to steel although lower than gray cast iron. The damping capacity of steel, S.G. iron and gray iron may be taken in the ratio of 1:1.8:5[27].

Corrosion Resistance: In most cases, the corrosion resistance of S.G. iron is similar to that of gray iron. Compared with carbon steel, it has superior corrosion resistance to attack by atmosphere, sea water, alkalies and some weak acids.

Wear Resistance: S.G. iron has outstanding wear resistance. The spheroidal graphite acts as reservoir to store lubricant for starting-up periods and to prevent galling and scuffing during periods of lubricant failure. Its wear resistance is equal to that of the best grades of gray iron and superior to that of carbon steel.

Magnetic Properties: The magnetic properties of S.G. iron is better than gray iron as change in graphite shape from flake to the nodular form results in an increase in magnetic permeability. Further improvement can be obtained with a ferritic matrix.

Thermal Shock Resistance: Ferritic S.G. iron can be heated to temperatures above 705° C, and drastically quenched in cold water without cracking.

High Temperature Service Properties: At high temperatures, gray irons suffer from structural changes and gas penetration and the consequent internal oxidation resulting in physical growth. S.G. irons are much more stable at high temperatures since the graphite spheroids are isolated from each other and do not provide paths for the penetration of gases as do the flakes. Surface oxidation of S.G. iron is also less. The creep strength of S.G. iron is also notably good.

6.5.3 Foundry Properties

No other ferrous material can equal the unusual combination of castability and mechanical properties of S.G. iron. It combines the main process advantages of gray irons like low melting point, good fluidity and castability for wide range of section thicknesses on accounts of having similar compositions in terms of carbon and silicon contents. However, S.G. irons solidify according to a mechanism quite different from gray cast irons. The solidification of such irons takes place with liquid and solid metal present throughout the casting and a very wide solidification temperature range is encountered. The solidification shrinkage and risering requirement of such irons are therefore different than gray irons.

6.5.4 Applications of S.G. Irons

The applications of S.G. irons are numerous and can be found almost in every branch of industry. By virtue of its versatile properties. S.G. iron has not only found extensive applications of its own castings but has also replaced not only the other types of ferrous castings but the steel forgings in many applications. The following can be taken as proportions of its applications[45]:

Applications		*% of total*
Spun Pipes	–	40%
Automotive Castings	–	25 to 30%
Machine Tool Castings	–	15-30%
Ingot Moulds	–	15%

As obvious from the above figures, the main application of S.G. iron in the highly industrialized countries is the manufacture of spun pipes. Before advent of this material the metal specified for such applications were gray cast iron and carbon steel. However, the mechanical properties of gray iron are lower than those of steel while the corrosion resistance of steel is poor as compared with that of gray iron. S.G. iron combines the corrosion resistance properties of gray iron with the mechanical properties of steel and thus is an obvious choice for spun pipes used for handling water, gas and petroleum products.

The second major field of application of S.G. iron is as automobile castings such as crank shafts, cylinder liners, piston rings, exhaust manifolds etc. Cars, trucks, tractors and other commercial vehicles and parts are the other main consumers of the S.G. iron castings.

The outstanding wear resistance of S.G. irons has led to its application as crank shafts, metal working rolls, punch dies, sheet metal dies, gears etc. The remainder of the S.G. iron castings may be referred to as general engineering castings for applications in iron and steel plants, railways and other fields. Metal working rolls, table rollers, ingot moulds, railway axle boxes and bearing shells etc. are some of such examples. Other applications are parts of pumps and compressors, construction machinery, paper industries machinery, power transmission equipment, mandrels, switch gear, brackets, couplings, street furniture, tunnel segments etc.

6.6 FOUNDRY PRACTICE

This includes usual operations of a foundry practice including melting and pouring, moulding and casting, gating and risering, cleaning etc. and heat treatment.

6.6.1 Melting and Pouring

The details of the melting practice adopted for production of S.G. iron castings have been already provided in the section 6.2.1.2.

The pouring temperatures of the metal obtained from different types of furnaces used are usually higher so as to take care of the heat losses incurred during magnesium treatment and post inoculation. The melt superheat also depends on the section thickness of the casting to be poured. The metal is quickly poured after magnesium treatment and post inoculation to minimize the effect of fading and depending on section thickness of the casting, the mould is usually poured at a temperature in the range of 1400 to 1480° C.

6.6.2 Moulding and Casting

The technology of moulding and casting of S.G. iron castings is similar to that of gray iron castings of similar size and quantities. The most common moulding and casting processes employed are green and dry sand moulding, shell moulding, CO_2-silicate/sand process and centrifugal casting. Most S.G. iron castings are made in green or dry sand moulds. Moulding sands used are also similar to those for gray iron castings but the moisture is carefully controlled because the S.G. iron melt having treated with magnesium oxidizes easily. The total combustible material in sands is usually limited to 6 to 7%. For large scale production, use of high pressure moulding giving dense and strong mould capable of preventing mould wall movement is finding increasing use.

6.6.3 Gating and Risering

Since S.G. iron is readily oxidizable, so a gating system which will minimize turbulence is used. Arrangement for retaining the slag and dirt in the gating system is very much needed and the metal should enter the mould with as little turbulence as possible. Generally, positive pressurized gating system with gating ratio of 4:8:3 are used. The optimum pouring time can be obtained with the equation as given below.

$$\text{Pouring Time (t)} = 0.65\sqrt{\text{pouring weight}}$$

Usually the metal should enter the bottom of the mould cavity through a sufficient number of in gates so that a minimum amount of metal flows from each gate. It is also desirable to provide runners with a height equal to twice the width. The total ingate area is function of the pouring weight and the pouring time.

Risering of S.G. iron is more difficult than gray iron due to its different solidification mode. S.G. iron does not freeze in skin forming manner as do most gray irons and steels. The solidification takes place with pasty zone throughout over a large temperature range. This, makes feeding difficult and depending on composition, dispersed shrinkage porosity may result. Generally, large risers and with a lot of risers are required to feed S.G. iron castings properly.

The danger of mould wall movement is much more pronounced in S.G. iron than gray iron and the need of a very stable and strong mould is very much there. However, less risering is needed in hypereutectic irons cast in dry sand moulds.

The cleaning and finishing operations used for S.G. iron castings are similar to those used for gray iron castings. However, removal of gates, risers etc. is not so easy because of the ductility and toughness of these castings.

6.6.4 Heat Treatment of S.G. Iron Castings

Some S.G. iron castings are used as-cast but great majority of them are heat treated. This is because a very wide range of properties can be obtained by controlling the compositions, foundry operations and/or heat treatment given. A variety of matrix structures can be obtained varying from all ferrite, ferrite and pearlite, all pearlite, martensite, tempered martensite or banite and in some special alloys, containing carbides or an austenitic matrix.

The main heat treatments given include :

6.6.4.1 Stress Relieving

This is used to reduce residual casting stresses such as those in complex castings in as-cast state or after normalizing. It is obtained by holding the casting at 535 to 620° C for one hour, plus one hour per inch of the section thickness. There is no marked structural change during this treatment although some softening occurs when high temperatures are used. Both cooling and heating rates should not be high during stress relieving otherwise cracks may form or stresses may be induced.

6.6.4.2 *Full Annealing or Ferritizing Anneal*

It is used to develop maximum ductility and best machinability. There are several methods which may be used. One typical heat treatment cycle includes heating to 850 to 950°, holding at this temperature for one hour plus one hour or more per inch of section thickness, cooling to 690° C uniformly and then holding at this temperature for 8 to 12 hours in total depending on section thickness.

6.6.4.3 *Normalizing*

It is used to obtain a homogenous structure of fine pearlite. A typical heat treatment cycle includes heating to 850 to 950° C, holding at this temperature for a minimum of one hour (depending on carbide present in the structure) and cooling to 785° C in furnace and then quenching in air. The heavier castings should contain alloying elements like Ni, Mo and Mn for satisfactory normalizing.

6.6.4.4 *Normalizing and Tempering*

Normalizing is commonly followed by tempering to reduce hardness and relieve residual stresses developed during rapid cooling in air. The tempering is carried by heating to 400 to 550° C for one hour.

6.6.4.5 *Quenching and Tempering*

This is given to obtain higher hardness and strength. Castings may be heated to between 850 to 950° C for austentizing followed by quenching in oil, water or brine and then heating for tempering in the temperature range of 300 to 600° C for periods of one hour + one hour per inch section thickness. The oil is preferred to water or brine.

6.6.4.6 Surface Hardening (Flame or Induction Hardening)

This treatment is used for obtaining high surface hardness and therefore high wear resistance. A pearlitic structure is desired before such treatment for maximum hardness and wear resistance. The hardness in the range of 53 to 60 R_c may be obtained. After flame hardening, it may be desirable to again stress relief the castings by heating at 150 to 200° C. Induction hardening is also used. High frequency current is used when shallow heating (to obtain thin case) is desired. Intermediate or low frequency current are used when superheating is desired. The water is used as quenching media although oil, brine or even compressed air may be also used.

Besides the above heat treatments, austempering and martenpering are also used similar to those used for steel heat treatment.

Compacted (Vermicular) Graphite Irons and Foundry Practice

7.1 INTRODUCTION

Compacted Graphite (CG) Iron has received considerable attention as an important engineering material in the past few years, even though it has been recognized for three decades or more. It is since 1965 that this iron has occupied its place as an important member of the family of cast irons with distinct properties requiring special manufacturing technologies. Compacted graphite irons are irons that exhibit graphite morphology intermediate to the interconnected flake graphite in gray cast irons and the spheroidal graphite in ductile cast irons. Compacted graphite, when observed under an optical microscope, appears as thickened flakes with rounded ends. It is therefore also called as VERMICULAR GRAPHITE (VG) and both the terms have been generally accepted for this intermediate form of the graphite.

Vermicular graphite thus represents a transition form from the stand point of compactness between flake and spheroidal graphite which is characterized by a low length (l) to thickness (t) ratio. The l/g ratio is generally between 2 and 10 and therefore much smaller than that of flake graphite ($l/g > 50$) but larger compared to that of spheroidal graphite ($l/g = 1$). In literature, this form of graphite is variously called[45] as type "P" graphite, "P_{441}" graphite, "quasi-flake" Form III, pseudo-lamellar, "chunky graphite", melko-plastin "catyjgrafit" etc. The mechanical properties of compacted graphite irons are strongly dependent on the shape, size and compactness of their graphite. It is well known that such cast irons are noticeable for their outstanding strength having a higher tensile strength, and particularly, a higher elongation than gray cast irons.

7.2. PRODUCTION OF COMPACTED GRAPHITE IRONS

Compacted graphite irons may be produced by several modification processes resulting in intermediate graphite forms of various compactness. In the present state of knowledge, the main ways for obtaining vermicular graphite are[45-48] :

1. Intensive desulphurization of the pig iron, particularly with calcium (leading to sulfur content < 0.002%) followed by rapid solidification in the mould.
2. Treatment of the base iron with small amounts of spheroidization promoting elements such as Mg or Ce to achieve incomplete modification.
3. Treatment of the base iron with both the spheroidizing and antispheroidizing elements e.g., Mg or Mg and Ce with Ti.
4. Treatment of the base iron with elements like Zr, Pb, Sb, Bi which under special conditions, can cause formation of vermicular graphite.

The influence of various elements on graphite morphology in the Fe-C-Si system is quite diverse with the absolute influence of any element being dependent on the presence of other elements and the cooling rate of the iron.

More or less similar steps are involved in the production of CG irons as used in case of SG irons i.e. production of base irons of suitable compositon followed by melt treatment and/or post inoculation of the treated melt.

7.2.1 Chemical Composition of CG Irons

The properties of CG irons are dependent on chemical composition which varies over a wide range of carbon equivalent (CE) values extending from hypoeutectic (CE = 3.7) to hypereutectic (CE = 4.7) with carbon contents of 3.1 to 4.0% and silicon in amounts of 1.7 to 3.0%. At constant silicon levels, a lower CE increases the chilling tendency and results in lower nodularity of graphite. At constant CE, higher silicon increases the nodularity of graphite. Hence, the optimum carbon and silicon contents have to be selected. The optimum CE is also a function of the section size of the casting. For a given section size, too high a CE will result in graphite flotation, while too low a CE may result in increased chilling tendency. For section thickness ranging from 10 to 40 mm, a eutectic composition (CE = 4.3%) is recommended to obtain optimum casting properties.

The manganese content can vary between 0.1 and 0.6%, while phosphorus content should be less than 0.06% in order to take the advantage of the ductility of this iron. Although CG irons have been produced from base irons having sulfur contents as high as 0.07 to 0.12%, it is more economical to desulfurize the iron to a level of 0.01 to 0.025% before the melt treatment is carried out since the higher the sulfur content of the base iron, the greater the amount of the treatment alloy required.

7.2.2 Melting

The melting furnaces used for preparation of base iron are induction furnaces, cupolas and arc furnaces and found to be sufficient to cater to the need of CG irons. Like S.G. irons, similar requirements of raw materials, superheating and desulfurization before the melt treatment for modification in the structure also apply. If a ferritic as-cast structure is desired, a pure pig iron with low manganese, phosphorus and sulfur contents is recommended. If some pearlite in the as-cast structure is acceptable, steel scrap can be used.

7.2.3 Melt Treatment and Treatment Alloys

The various methods of melt treatment for modification of the structure of the base iron have been already outlined in the section 7.2. The compositions of typical treatment alloys used in the production of CG iron are given in the Table 7.1.

CG iron can be obtained like S.G. iron by treating with magnesium iron-silicon alloy (Type 1). The residual magnesium content is controlled in the range of 0.013 to 0.022%. A better control of residual magnesium can be achieved if In-Mould treatment process is used. In case sulfur content of the base iron is high, higher residual magnesium content will be necessary.

The alloys containing spheroidizing or compactizing elements balanced by anticompactizing elements like Ti have much wider industrial application. For example, the treatment alloy type 2 containing 5% Mg and 0.3% Ce balanced by 9% Ti is used in order to obtain 0.015 to 0.035% residual Mg, 0.06 to 0.13% residual Ti and low levels of Ce in the final cast iron. This treatment alloy

TABLE 7.1: NOMINAL COMPOSITIONS OF TYPICAL TREATMENT ALLOYS FOR CG IRON[48]

Alloy Number	*Alloy Type*	*Composition %*							*Neutral Elements*	
		Spheroidizing or Compactizing Elements					*Anticompactizing Elements*			
		Mg	*Ce*	*La*	*TRE**	*Ca*	*Ti*	*Al*	*Si*	*Fe*
1.	Mg-Fe-Si alloy	5	–	–	–	1	–	< 1.2	45	Balance
2.	Mg-Fe-Si-Ti alloy	5	0.3	–	0.3	< 1	9	< 1.5	52	Balance
3.	Mg-Fe-Si-Ti-Ca alloy	5	0.3	–	0.3	4.5	9	1.2	50	Balance
4.	Ce-Fe-Si-Ca-La alloy	–	24	14.4	48	7.5	–	4.3	33.2	Balance
5.	Rare earth alloy	–	30	50	80	–	–	–	–	Balance
6.	Rare earth alloy	–	16	80	96	–	–	–	–	Balance
7.	Rare earth alloy	–	2.9	26.5	29.4	0.63	–	–.13	30.5	Balance
8.	Mg-rare earth-FeSi alloy	3.7	0.8	0.5	1.7	1.05	–	0.88	45.3	Balance
9.	Mg-rare earth-FeSi alloy	4.3	0.7	1.8	2.9	0.66	–	0.90	45.3	Balance

TRE* = Total Rare Earth Elements

was later improved by the inclusion of 4 to 5.5% Ca (alloy type 3) to extend the working range of residual magnesium and the tolerable range of base sulfur. A wide range of carbon and silicon contents (3.15 to 4% C and 1.7 to 3% Si) can be used to produce CG iron in section thicknesses of 12 to 65 mm. The base iron for this iron can have sulfur contents in the range of 0.02 to 0.04% resulting in final sulfur levels of 001 to 0.02%. The amount of magnesium-titanium alloy used is not critical but depends on the base sulfur content.

The type 4 alloy can also be included in the above category of alloy. Additions of 0.2% of this alloy resulted in CG structures in castings ranging in section thickness from 25 to 127 mm but castings showed a rather high chilling tendency.

The treatment of the base iron with rare earth alloys (e.g. type 5 alloy) was one of the first processes to gain industrial application. This alloy containing cerium and mischmetal is used for production of medium and heavy section CG iron castings. The residual Ce contents of 0.013 to 0.075% are required depending on base sulfur content. Although treatment with such alloy containing rare earth offers a number of advantages over magnesium treatment such as lower fading time and no smoke formation during reaction time, there is a serious problem of showing high chilling tendency in thin section castings.

Rare earth alloys containing a higher lanthanum/rare earth ratio than typical mish metal have been suggested (alloys 6 & 7) to alleviate the chilling tendency. However, post inoculation is required when silicon-free alloys are used.

Another way to avoid the chilling tendency associated with mischmetal treatment is to use a Mg-rare earth-FeSi type alloy (alloy 8 & 9). When these alloys are used in conjunction with the In-Mould process, a residual Mg, Ce and La content of 0.018 to 0.028% was required to get CG iron structure when the base sulfur was 0.016%.

Another approach for producing CG iron is to substitute Al for most of the silicon in the iron. This has the advantages of allowing the use of a magnesium-ferro silicon alloy because aluminium has an anticompactizing effect and can counter balance the influence of magnesium. This idea has been applied using both the ladle and in-mould treatment using 5% magnesium-ferrosilicon alloy with 0.3% Ce and with the aluminium levels of 2.68 to 4.98%. No post inoculation was required.

Treatment Temperature: Regardless of the treatment alloy used for a specific alloy addition and base sulfur content, there is an optimum range of treatment temperatures. For example, for an iron with base sulfur of 0.12 to 0.13% and a treatment addition of 1.75% alloy, the treatment temperature must be between 1468 to 1510° C. Too low a temperature results in increased nodularity and an excessive temperature causes premature alloy dissolution and iron obtained is gray iron with flake graphite.

7.2.4 Post Inoculation

It is generally found that CG iron exhibits a high chilling tendency, especially in sections thinner than 6 mm. To counteract this negative effect, it is necessary to use either silicon in the treatment alloy or some type of post inoculation. Most of the time, 0.2 to 0.3% ferrosilicon containing 75% Si is used for post inoculation. Nevertheless in thin section castings, it is difficult to counteract the chilling tendency by post inoculation. It has been suggested that 0.1 to 0.2% Al or a Ferrosilicon-Ti-Al alloy of suitable composition can be used as post inoculants to take care of such problems.

7.2.5 Moulding and Casting

Like S.G. iron castings, all types of moulding materials that can produce rigid moulds can be used for making CG castings. Such moulding materials may include bentonite-bonded, cement-bonded and resin-bonded sands.

CG iron melts are more sensitive to sulfur pick-up from the mould than are SG iron melts. Therefore, CG iron must not be overtreated. Particular attention should be payed when using reclaimed resin-bonded sands containing para-toluosulfonic acid (PTS) as a hardening catalyst. There is a great danger of sulfur pick-up in such cases of mould materials. It may be useful to substitute phosphoric acid in part for PTS as a hardener when using such mould materials. Also, the application of protective mould coatings with lime, magnesia or talc base is recommended.

7.2.6 Mechanism of Vermicular Graphite Formation

Several authors have proposed mechanisms for formation of vermicular graphite but very few are in agreement[46,50]. The hypotheses vary from the growth of graphite being in contact with the liquid to graphite growth occurring due to partial dissolution of the austenite shell surrounding a graphite spheroid. The presence of a highly surface active element like titanium in contact with graphite particles is believed to prevent formation of graphite spheroids and to promote the formation of the standard form - compacted. Its adsorption on the graphite surface opposes the effect of magnesium. The modification brought about is first manifest as rounding of the ends of graphite flakes followed by general thickening and shortening of the graphite resulting in the flakes becoming very compact while remaining interconnected within a eutectic cell.

7.3 STRUCTURE AND CLASSIFICATION OF COMPACTED OR VERMICULAR GRAPHITE

As earlier mentioned, vermicular or compacted graphite irons are irons that exhibit a graphite morphology intermediate to the interconnected, flake graphite in the gray cast iron and the isolated spheroidal graphite in ductile cast iron (Fig. 7.1). Compacted graphite, when observed in two dimensions under an optical microscope, appears as thickened flakes with rounded ends (Fig. 7.1b). The three-dimensional views of compacted graphite, as revealed by SEM examination of deeply etched samples, reveal interconnected graphite within the eutectic cell similar to flakes but more compacted in nature (Fig. 7.2). In fact, the graphite does not appear as flakes but rather as clusters. It is short, stubby and irregular in nature having rounded edges as seen under the optical microscope.

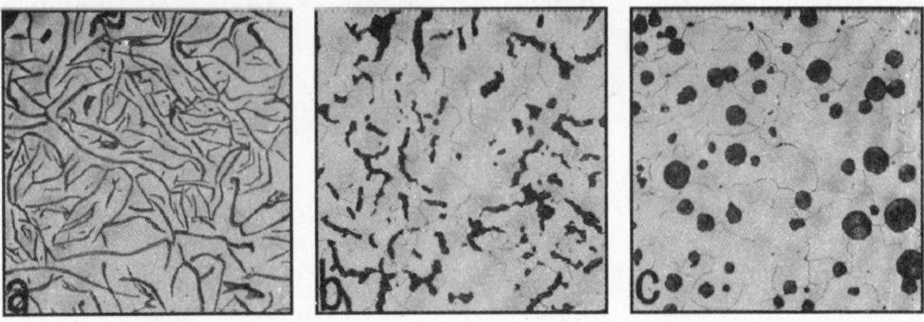

Fig. 7.1: Comparison of various shapes of graphite in different irons (a) Flake graphite, (b) Vermicular graphite, (c) Spheroidal graphite (From J. Sissener *et al.*,AFS Cast Metals Research Journal, Vol. 8, 1972, p. 179).

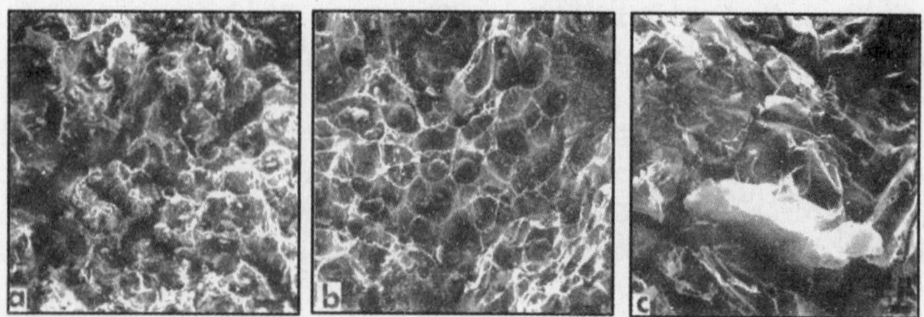

Fig. 7.2: SEM views (a & b) of full deep etch of examples of graphite in CG irons (Reprinted with permission of ASM International).

Several efforts have been made to provide classifications for the diverse forms of graphite found in castings of such irons[46,51,52]. ASTM has one classification in which vermicular or compacted shapes of graphite are designated as ASTM P-graphite. Another classification proposed by L. Sofroni et al. distinguishes intermediate forms of graphite based on the length, thickness and length-to-thickness ratio of the graphite. Still another classification proposed by the Ductile Iron Society (DIS) includes nine types of graphite. However, most of the published properties of CG irons appear to have contained Sofroni Type III graphite, which is similar to ASTM Type P and DIS Type VII.

7.4 PROPERTIES OF V.G. IRONS

7.4.1 Engineering Properties

Mechanical Properties: The mechanical properties of CG iron depends on a number of factors such as composition, structure (nodularity of compacted graphite and matrix) and the section size governing the cooling rate. The typical range of room temperature properties for CG irons with ferritic and perlitic matrices are given in Table 7.2.

The yield point ratio (ratio of yield strength to tensile strength) of CG irons ranges from 0.72 to 0.82 which is higher than for SG iron of the same composition. Thus, they have a higher loading capacity.

The average tensile strength to hardness ratio of gray iron is 1.3, compared with 2.08 for CG iron and 2.75 for SG iron. The intermediate mechanical behaviour of CG iron is quite apparent. The CG iron shows a good degree of deformation compared to gray iron. For example, CG iron shows elongation to the extent of ~ 8% whereas elongation of gray iron is hardly measurable. The microfractography of CG iron (Fig. 7.3a) at 240X is similar to that of SG iron[53] (Fig. 7.3b) : a ductile honeycomb fracture which embraces the graphite particles. On the other hand, gray iron shows a brittle fracture.

TABLE 7.2: TYPICAL MECHANICAL PROPERTIES OF CG IRONS

Properties	*Matrix*	
	Ferritic	*Pearlitic*
Tensile strength	36 to 55,000 psi (248 to 380 N/mm^2)	59 to 90,000 psi (407 to 621 N/mm^2)
0.2% offset Yield strength	25 to 43,000 psi (172 to 300 N/mm^2)	45 to 63,000 psi (310 to 434 N/mm^2)
Elongation	3 to 8%	1 to 3%
Hardness	130 to 179 BHN	207 to 269 BHN
Modulus of Elasticity	17500 to 18300,000 psi (121300 to 126200 N/mm^2)	18500 to 24000,000 psi (127200 to 166000 N/mm^2)

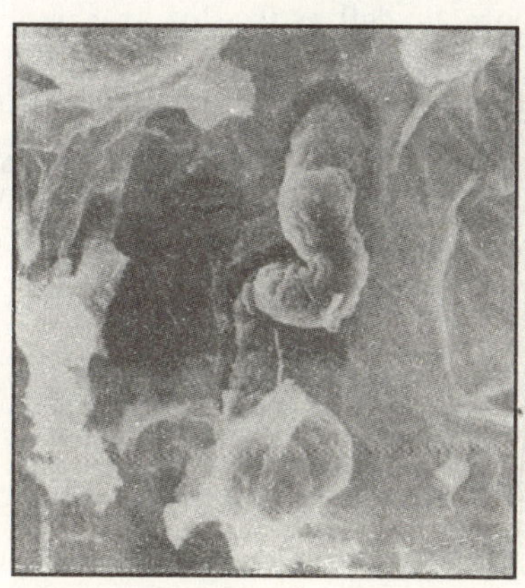

(a)

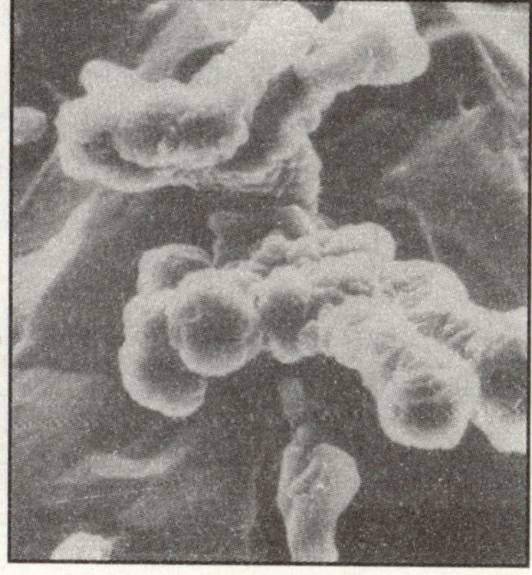

(b)

Fig. 7.3: Fractographs of different cast irons, at 240X, (a) CG iron & (b) SG iron

Both the pearlite/ferrite ratio (which can be increased by alloying or heat treatment) and the nodularity of graphite influence the mechanical properties of CG iron. The tensile strength and elongation increase as the nodularity of CG irons increases. The tensile strength, yield strength and hardness of CG iron increase with an increasing pearlite/ferrite ratio, whereas elongation decreases.

The ultimate compressive strength of predominantly pearlitic CG iron is approximately three times the tensile strength. The SG irons exhibit substantially greater toughness than CG irons at low pearlite contents but the pearlitic CG irons have impact strengths equivalent to those of SG irons.

The mechanical properties of CG irons are less sensitive to section thickness of the casting than are those of gray irons. The variation with the temperature of tensile strength, yield strength and elongation of CG iron is found to be similar to that of SG iron but the values are somewhat lower. On the other hand, the growth and scaling of CG irons at high temperature was found to be not significantly different from those of gray irons of similar composition.

Thermal Conductivity: The thermal conductivity of CG iron is very close to that of gray iron and considerably higher than that of SG iron. This may be attributed to its similar interconnectivity of graphite structure within the eutectic cell as that of gray iron.

Corrosion Resistance: The corrosion resistance of CG iron at room temperature in sulfuric acid is found to be nearly half that of gray iron but with increasing temperature the difference becomes smaller. The pearlitic matrix shows a higher corrosion resistance than the ferritic one.

Machinability: In general, for a given matrix, the machinability of CG iron is between that of gray and SG iron.

Damping Capacity: The relative damping capacity of gray iron, CG iron and SG iron lies in the ratio of 1.0 : 0.6 : 0.34.

7.4.2 Foundry Properties

Fluidity: The CG iron has an intermediate position with respect to fluidity between the gray iron (which shows best fluidity) and the SG iron (showing worst fluidity). However, because CG irons are stronger than gray irons with the same carbon equivalent (CE), a higher CE can be used to obtain the same strength, allowing greater fluidity and easier pouring of thin sections.

Shrinkage Characteristics: To get sound castings of CG irons free from shrinkage porosity is easier than those of SG irons and slightly more difficult than those of gray irons. CG iron castings show low shrinkage and therefore can sometimes be cast without the need for a riser. In many cases, the same running and feeding systems could be used to produce sound castings of CG irons as used for gray iron castings[54]. The CG iron solidifies with an intermediate outward expansion force and thus it requires less feeding than SG iron castings made in any type of mould.

Casting Yield: The yields for large castings of CG irons vary between 65 to 75% depending on casting complexity and weight.

Dross Formation: The problem of dross formation of CG iron castings is similar to that of SG iron castings and therefore the best conditions for producing dross free CG irons are the same as recommended for SG irons.

Chilling Tendency: The chilling tendency of CG irons is similar to that of gray irons.

7.5 APPLICATIONS OF CG IRONS

One serious limitation of gray iron is that it is a brittle material. Even in high strength gray iron, elongation is normally less than 1% which for many applications is insufficient. Replacement of gray iron with a material of higher strength, ductility and toughness such as S.G. iron is not always possible because of poorer casting properties, lower thermal conductivity, higher modulus of elasticity and so forth. In such cases, CG iron can close the gap between the two materials, because its mechanical properties are closer to those of SG iron, while its physical (expansion, conductivity) and elevated temperature properties (thermal fatigue, thermal shock) are closer to those of gray iron. Hence, the primary factor in the selection of CG iron for practical application is its position between gray and SG iron. CG iron can be used wherever tensile properties of high strength gray iron are insufficient or where the use of SG or malleable iron is not essential. From an economic view point, the casting technology of CG iron is much simpler than that of SG iron or malleable iron.

The examples of typical applications of CG irons are bed plates for large diesel engines, crank cases, gear-box and turbo charger housings, connecting forks, bearing brackets, pulleys for truck servo drives, sprocket wheels and eccentric gears.

Because of the fact that the thermal conductivity of CG iron is higher than that of SG iron, the former is preferred for castings operating at elevated temperatures and/or under thermal fatigue conditions. Such applications include ingot moulds, crank cases, cylinder heads, exhaust manifolds and brake disks.

8

High-Duty (High Strength) Cast Irons

8.1 INTRODUCTION

The definition of the term High-Duty Cast Irons in literature is quite vague and described variously by different authors. According to Rolfe and Laing[55], this term is used to describe two distinct classes of materials:

1. Those of high strength, such as can be obtained by improving the properties of the matrix, and controlling the graphite quantity, distribution, flake shape and size;
2. Those with some special characteristics, such as high resistance to corrosion or heat, where the enhanced properties are often due to the development of special structural constituents by means of additional alloys.

As described above, thus high-duty cast irons simply mean High-Strength Gray Irons and Special or Alloy Cast Irons. However, quite frequently, the term high-duty cast irons are used to refer the former class of irons i.e. high-strength irons, as also described by Rollason[56].

According to Metals Hard Book[57], the term High-Strength Irons refer to those irons which have tensile strength generally greater than 40,000 psi (i.e. > 20 tons/in^2 or 308.8 N/mm^2). This chapter will therefore be developed to production, characterization and applications of such high-strength gray cast irons.

High-strength irons are frequently known as pearlitic cast irons, since when properly constituted, they are composed chiefly of pearlite. The mechanical properties of such irons thus resemble somewhat that of steel having the eutectoid proportion of carbon except that a variation is naturally introduced by the presence of graphite inclusions. The strongest irons are thus being those in which the number and size of these graphite inclusions is a minimum and the grains of the pearlite ground mass is as fine as possible[55] (Fig. 8.1). Such irons show generally a high strength and a high resistance to wear, shock and heat. They are produced in practice by various distinct processes and some of these are proprietary.

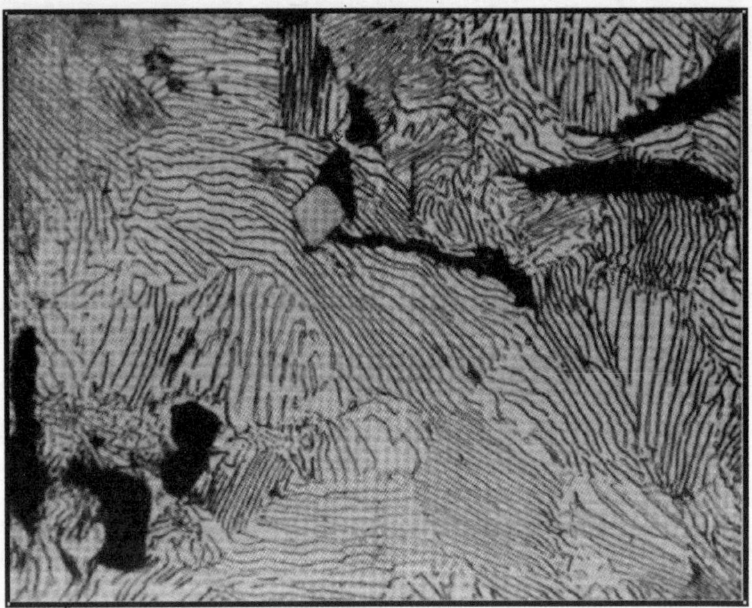

Fig. 8.1: Pearlitic high-strength gray iron showing graphite flakes in matrix of pearlite, X1000.

8.2 MANUFACTURE OF HIGH-STRENGTH GRAY IRONS

High-strength irons are manufactured by[55-58]:

1. The use of special melting and casting techniques
2. The addition of alloying elements

8.2.1 Manufacture by Use of Special Melting and Casting Techniques

Various processes used under the category of the first method of manufacture of such irons are based on the application of the following principles:

(*i*) Reducing the total carbon content and therefore graphite by using in the melting charge sufficient low carbon pig iron and steel scrap.
(*ii*) Adjustment of the carbon/silicon ratio to obtain minimum graphite without producing either free ferrite or free carbide.
(*iii*) Treatment of the molten iron with chemical agent like soda ash (Na_2CO_3) to reduce the phosphorus content (which is undesirable where high resistance to shock or heat is required).
(*iv*) Graphitizing a low-carbon and/or low silicon iron with a suitable ladle addition i.e. inoculation treatment of the melt.
(*v*) Combining inoculation treatment of above iron with minor additions of alloying elements like Cr, Mo and/or Ni.

Several of these processes not only aim at reducing the amount of graphite formed in such irons but also at the refining of the graphite. In this endevour, the low-carbon and/or low-silicon melt produced by careful charging and melting, which under normal casting additions may be mottled or white on freezing is so treated as to cause separation of the fine grained graphite and the casting is gray and machinable. The separation of fine graphite is effected by:

(*i*) Super heating the metal produced from cupola or other furnace so that on pouring into the mould, the latter gets preheated to a high temperature which retards cooling of the melt through the critical range.
(*ii*) Running excess metal through the mould to ensure mould preheating and retard cooling of the melt.
(*iii*) Preheating the mould to receive the metal poured at normal temperatures (This method has greater certainty and has thus obvious advantages over other methods).
(*iv*) Treating the metal poured with the addition of graphitizing compounds in the ladle (This method has much more exact control on graphite precipitation).

The following are some of the examples of the high-strength irons produced on the basis of the above methods.

8.2.1.1 Compositions, Properties and Applications of Unalloyed High-Strength Gray Irons

8.2.1.1.1 Lanj Perlit Iron

This iron is produced by pouring a low-silicon and preferably a low-carbon iron of predetermined composition and temperature in a preheated sand mould. This iron in which silicon may be as low as 0.5% would be normally white or mottled but by means of a suitable balance between composition and mould temperature, a controlled quantity of finely dispersed graphite is produced so as to give iron of tensile strength of 20 to 22 tons/in^2 (308.8 to 338.8 N/mm^2) and of consistent quality both in light and heavy sections. The mould temperature regulates graphitization in the light sections and the silicon content that in heavy sections. The slow and controlled cooling involved by casting in a hot mould avoids the setting up of contraction stresses such as are inseparable from casting in a cold mould. The iron produced is thus very suitable for the manufacture of Diesel engine cylinder liners and pistons without requiring a stress-relieving treatment.

The irons produced by the Lanz Process in which silicon percentage may be made very low, show little growth at higher temperatures and are especially suitable for use under oxidizing conditions which promote growth. The physical growth of the casting increases in proportion to the silicon content of the iron. The quality of low growth of the above iron has thus led to a number of applications of this iron such as retorts for low temperature carbonization, fire bars, ingot moulds and like where good heat resistance is required.

The typical composition of the Lanz Perlit Iron is :

Combined carbon	–	0.85%
Graphitic carbon	–	2.25%
Total carbon	–	3.10%
Silicon	–	0.80%
Sulfur	–	0.135%
Phosphorus	–	0.22%
Manganese	–	1.08%.

8.2.1.1.2 Thyssen-Emmel Iron

This is another pearlitic iron of high strength, being superior to Lanz Perlit in this respect. The Emmel iron can be made with a tensile strength in the range of 23 to 27 tons/in^2 (354.2 to 415.8 N/mm^2). This iron has, however, a much higher silicon content and is therefore not comparable with Perlit where resistance to heat is required in service. Again, it shows much greater variation in different parts of the casting. In order to make a stronger iron, the carbon content is reduced to a low figure by using some 50% or more of the steel scrap in the furnace charge with the corresponding adjustment of the cupola blast conditions. It is essential to use a high casting temperature. The iron is cast without any particular difficulty but has somewhat high shrinkage and thus requiring the use of carefully designed riser. For castings of thin sections, Thyssen-Emmel iron is clearly superior to Lanj Perlit but being inferior for casting of heavy sections or for those where shock of heat may be experienced in service.

The typical analysis of this iron is as follows:

Combined carbon	–	0.75%
Graphitic carbon	–	2.00%
Total carbon	–	2.75%
Silicon	–	2.60%
Sulfur	–	0.10%
Phosphorus	–	0.15%
Manganese	–	1.50%

8.2.1.1.3 Inoculated Cast Irons

These ions are obtained by the addition to the molten iron in the ladle of a suitable proportion of the graphitizer (inoculant) just prior to casting. The basis iron to which the addition is made should have a controlled and comparatively low carbon content i.e. between 2.4 and 3%. The silicon content is also lower than that required to produce normal gray iron castings. The deficiency in silicon content is made up by the addition of a controlled amount of Fe-Si or other graphitizer in proportion to the carbon content. The graphite is caused to separate as flake which however is not of the conventional coarse form but is comparatively fine and distributed randomly in the matrix. Such irons of finely dispersed graphite in a pearlite matrix are considerable stronger than ordinary gray irons and can be made of tensile strength from 20 tons/in^2 (308.8 N/mm^2) upwards while this strength can be further enhanced by additional alloying elements such as Cu, Mo, Ni etc.

There are two proprietary processes of manufacture of inoculated irons depending on the application of a particular inoculant as given below.

Meehanite Process: In this process, calcium silicide is the inoculant used. The term mechanite is the proprietary name for the irons produced by the above process. Meehanite iron is made in a number of grades and an approximate composition range of such irons for high strength purposes is as follows :

Total carbon	–	2.40 to 2.70%
Silicon	–	1.10 to 1.50%
Sulfur	–	0.05 to 0.14%
Phosphorus	–	0.10 to 0.20%
Manganese	–	0.65 to 1.00%

Such irons have tensile strength of 20 to 25 tons/in^2 (308.8 to 385 N/mm^2) with BHN in the range of 260 to 300 and the iron is readily machinable.

Ni-Tensyl Process: The graphitizing additions for this process are Fe-Si and Nickel shot. Such irons are frequently melted in cupolas and the charge contains from 50 to 90% steel scrap with the remaining material consisting of Ni-tensyl scrap and selected ordinary scrap or pig iron. The composition range and properties of such irons are:

Total carbon	–	2.5 to 3.0%
Silicon	–	0.5 to 0.8%
Sulfur	–	0.12% max.
Phosphorus	–	0.20% max.
Manganese	–	0.7 to 1.0%
Tensile strength	–	22 to 30 tons/in^2 (338.8 to 462 N/mm^2)
BHN	–	280 to 300

By inoculation in the ladle, the silicon content is increased to 1.25 to 1.75% and the nickel content lies in the range of 1.0 to 2.0%. Such composition gives satisfactory results over a wide range of casting section thickness.

8.2.2 Manufacture by Addition of Alloying Elements

The tensile strength of gray cast irons can be also significantly increased by minor additions of some alloying elements like Ni, Cr, Cu and Mo singly or in combination.

Small additions of Cr upto about 0.5 to 0.75% cause significant increase in strength of gray iron mainly by promoting formation of pearlite. Cr is a carbide promoter and in light section castings or at heavy addition rates, it can cause chill formation. It is normally added as a ferrochromium alloy and care should be taken to ensure that this alloy is completely dissolved.

Nickel additions of upto 2% cause only a minor increase in the tensile strength of gray iron. It has a minor graphitizing effect and is less powerful than silicon in this respect. However, on high contents, it hardens the iron as it produces grain refinement of pearlite and thus increases the strength properties. It is normally added as elemental material.

Small additions of molybdenum (in the range of 0.25 to 0.75%) have a significant impact on the strength of gray iron. This is the result of matrix strengthening and refinement of graphite flakes. It is normally added as a ferromolybdenum alloy.

Copper also increases the tensile strength of gray iron by promoting formation of pearlite matrix. It is normally added in amounts of 0.25 to 0.5%. It has a mild graphitizing effect and therefore does not promote carbides in light sections.

Besides the above elements which are commonly added to produce high-strength gray irons, small additions of tin (in the range of 0.025 to 0.1%) as well as that of vanadium have been also found to be beneficial in increasing the strength of gray irons.

Usually, unalloyed high strength gray irons have tensile strength upto 24 tons/in^2 (369.6 N/mm^2) and alloyed ones upto 40 tons/in^2 (616 N/mm^2).

The following are examples of alloyed high-strength gray irons which find different applications in foundry industry.

8.2.2.1 Compositions, Properties and Applications of Alloyed High-Strength Gray Irons

8.2.2.1.1 Pearlitic Irons

Alloyed gray irons containing 1/2-2% Ni and Cr upto 0.8% and Mo upto 0.6% are used for many general engineering castings. The addition of Sn in amounts upto 0.1% promotes formation of a fully pearlitic matrix.

High carbon Ni-Cr-Mo gray cast iron is useful for resisting thermal shock in applications such as die casting moulds and brake-drums. Both the Ni and Cr help in refinement of the matrix whereas Mo strengthens the matrix. Cr (0.6%) - Mo (0.6%) irons are useful for engine liners, press sleeves, dies etc. where wear resistance in heavy sections is desired. Gray irons having 1% each of Cr and Mo are used for piston-ring pots.

8.2.2.1.2 Acicular Irons

With the correct amounts of Ni and Mo correlated with the cooling rate of a particular casting, the pearlitic change point can be suppressed and an acicular intermediate constituent (ferrite needles in austenite matrix i.e. Bainite) can be produced with high mechanical properties. Such acicular gray cast iron (Fig. 8.2) is

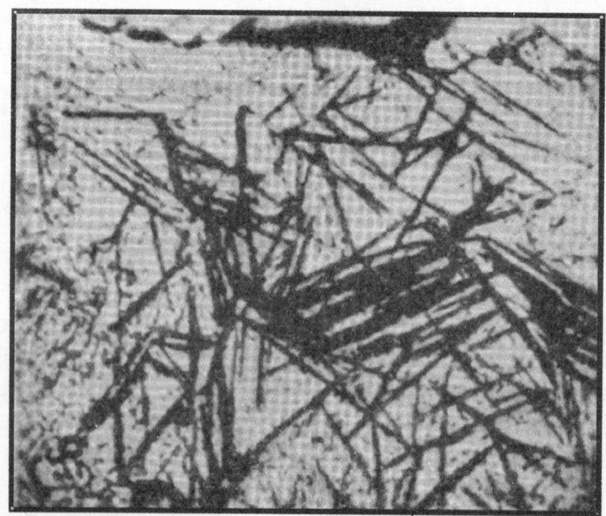

Fig. 8.2: Acicular gray cast iron showing dark-etching needles, X1000[55]

very much tougher than any of the pearlitic cast irons of lower strength. The tensile strength of such acicular irons with a carbon content of about 3% will vary from 25 to 35 tons/in^2 (380 to 540 N/mm^2).

Acicular irons will have carbon in the range of 2.9 to 3.2%, nickel in the range of 1.5 to 2% and Mo from 0.3 to 0.6%. The copper can replace Ni upto 1.5%. The phosphorus content should not exceed 0.15% in presence of Mo as being detrimental to matrix. Quite large variation in silicon content can be tolerated but Cr in excess of 0.5% is harmful. Such rigid, high-strength shock resisting irons are used for Diesel crank shaft, gears etc. However, these irons should not be used at temperatures higher than 300° C as the structure changes rapidly at 600 to 750° C.

References

1. J.J. Moore, *Fundamentals of Foundry Technology* (ed. P.D. Webster), Portcullis Press Ltd., Surrey, 1980, p. 338.
2. H.J. Leyshon and R.B. Coates, BCIRA J., 1962, Vol. 10, p. 28.
3. L.F. Porter and P.C. Rosenthal, Trans. AFS, 1952, Vol. 60, p. 545.
4. J.E. Rehder, Brit. Foundrym., 1968, Vol. 61, p. 471.
5. H.J. Leyshon, ibid, 1966, Vol. 59, p. 49.
6. M.J. Selby, ibid, 1978, Vol. 71, p. 241.
7. S.F. Carter and F.T. Kaiser, Trans. AFS, 1986, Vol. 94, p. 809.
8. R.T. Taft, *Foundry Tr. J.*, 1974, Vol. 137, p. 707.
9. C.H. Wilson and W.J. Driscol, Brit. Foundrym., 1976, Vol. 69, p. 97.
10. Metals Handbook, Ninth Edition, *Casting*, Vol. 15, ASM Metals Park, Ohio, 1988, p. 383.
11. *The Cupola and its Operation*, 3rd edn., 1965, AFS, Illinois, p. 306.
12. V.H. Patterson and M.J. Lalich, *Foundry Technology*, Source Book, 1982, ASM & AFS, Metals Park, Ohio, p. 298.
13. A. Boyles, *The Structure of Cast Iron*, 1947, ASM.
14. B. Lux, AFS Trans., 1964, Vol. 72, p. 222.
15. S.R. Sampath and J.A. Ballard, Procd. Seminar on Cast Iron Today, 1970, Bombay, p. 32.
16. G.N. Rao and P.K. Gupta, *NML Tech. J.*, 1971, p. 19.
17. J.R. Nieman and L.W. McFarland, *US Patent* 3, 991808, No. 16, 1976.
18. *Metals Handbook on Casting*, Ninth edn., Volume 15, 1988, ASM, Metals Park, Ohio, p. 638.
19. J.T.H. Pearce and J.J. Dudley, *Fundamentals of Foundry Technology* (edr. P.D. Webster), 1980, Portcullis Press Ltd., Surrey, p. 229.
20. R. Soundararajan, Pro. Winter School on Advanced Foundry Technology, Deptt. of Metallurgical Engg., PSG College of Tech., Coimbatore, Nov. 5-17, 1979, p. 201.
21. Malleable Iron Castings, Malleable Founders Society, Cleveland, Ohio, 1960, p. 55 and 157.
22. J.T.H. Pearce and J.J. Dudley, *Fundamentals of Foundry Technology* (edr. P.D. Webster), 1980, Portcullis Press Ltd., Survey, p. 243 and p. 245.

91

23. H. Morrough, Trans. AFS, 1948, Vol. 56, p. 72.
24. H. Morrogh and W.J. Williams, J. *Iron & Steel Inst.*, 1948, Vol. 158, p. 306.
25. B.G. Sastry, *Indian Foundry J.*, 1968, Vol. 14, p. 39.
26. Pierre-Marie Ca banne and M. Gazne, *Indian Foundry J.*, 2006, Vol. 52, No. 3, p. 21.
27. R.N. Gandhi, Procd. Seminar on Cast Iron Today, Feb. 1970, Bombay, p. 129.
28. E.K. Modl, *The British Foundrym.*, 1970, Vol. 63, p. 193.
29. R.W. Heine, C.R. Loper and P.C. Rosenthal, *Principles of Metal Casting*, Tata McGraw-Hill Publishing Co. Ltd., New Delhi, 1976, p. 614.
30. Metals Handbook on Casting, Ninth Edn., Vol. 15, 1988, ASM, Metals Park, Ohio, p. 647.
31. W.E. Snow, *Foundry*, 1964, Vol. 92, p. 99.
32. R.F. Dalton, *Mod. Cast.*, 1965, Vol. 48, p. 50.
33. A.F.S. Committee 124, *Mod. Cast.* 1967, Vol. 52, p. 110.
34. B. Lux, *Cast. Met. Res. J.*, 1972, Vol. 8, p. 49.
35. B. Lux, ibid., p. 25.
36. B. Lux, F. Mollard and I. Minkoff, Proc. Second Int. Sym. on Metallurgy of Cast Irons, May 29-31, 1974, Geneva, Switzerland, p. 371.
37. J.T.H. Pearce and J.J. Dudley, *Fundamentals of Foundry Technology* (edr. P.D. Webster), 1980, Portcullis Press Ltd., Surrey, p. 250.
38. R. Hummer, Proc. Second Int. Sym. on Metallurgy of Cast Irons, May 29-31, 1974, Geneva, Switzerland, p. 147.
39. R.L. Snezhnov and A.A. Zhukov, ibid., p. 12.
40. R.H. McSwain and C.E. Bates, ibid., p. 423.
41. J.P. Sadocha and J.E. Gruzleski, ibid., p. 443.
42. S. Banerjee, *Brit. Foundrym.*, 1965, Vol. 58, p. 334.
43. A.A. Gorshkov, Russ. Cast. Prod., 1963, p. 164.
44. M.J. Lalich and J.R. Hitchings, AFS Trans., Vol. 84, p. 1276.
45. Procd. of National Seminar on Production Technology of S.G. Iron Castings, Oct. 11-12, 1979, Poona, Local Chapter, IIF, p. 27.
46. L. Safroni, I. Riposan and I. Chira, Proc. Second Int. Sym. on Metallurgy of Cast Irons, May 29-31, 1974, Geneva, Switzerland, p. 179.
47. G.F. Sergeant, *British Foundrym.*, 1978, Vol. 71, p. 115.
48. R.W. Monroe and C.E. Bates, AFS Trans., 1982, Vol. 90, p. 615.
49. *Metals Hand Book on Casting*, Ninth edn., Vol. 15, 1988, ASM, Metals Park, Ohio, p. 667.
50. K.P. Cooper and C.R. Loper Jr., AFS Trans., 1978, Vol. 86, p. 267.
51. C.K. Donoho, *Modern Cast.*, Vol. 39, 1961, p. 65.
52. W. Rhury, *AFS Cast Metals Res. J.*, Vol. 6, 1970, p. 153.
53. J. Sissener, W. Thury, R. Hummer and E. Nechtelberger, *AFS Cast Metals Res. J.*, Vol. 8, 1972, p. 178.
54. K.P. Cooper and C.R. Loper Jr., AFS Trans., Vol. 86, 1978, p. 241.
55. J. Laing and R.T. Rolfe, *A Manual of Foundry Practice for Cast Iron*, Chapman & Hall, London, 1960, p. 262.
56. E.C. Rollason, *Metallurgy for Engineers*, Edward Arnold (Publishers) Ltd., Hill Street (U.K.), 1973, p. 278.

57. Metals Handbook, (edr. T. Lyman), ASM, Metals Park, Ohio, 1948, p. 515.
58. H.T. Angus, *Cast Iron: Physical and Engineering Properties*, Butterworths, London, 1978, p. 176.
59. O.P. Khanna and M. Lal, *A Text Book of Foundry Technology*, Dhanpat Rai Publications (P) Ltd., New Delhi, 2001, p. 552.
60. Proceedings of Winter School on Advanced Foundry Technology, Deptt. of Metallurgical Engg., PSG College of Technology, Coimbatore, Nov. 5-7, 1979.